DIVERTICULITIS DIET AFTER 60

OVER 2100 DAYS OF HEALTHY & HIGH-FIBER RECIPES TO PREVENT FLARE-UPS AND BOOST YOUR DIGESTIVE HEALTH - INCLUDES A CUSTOM 31-DAY MEAL PLAN FOR SENIORS + 3 BONUSES

JEAN MORESBY

TABLE OF CONTENTS

INTRODUCTION

Welcome to Your Golden Years

Embarking on the golden years can bring a sense of freedom mixed with apprehension, especially when it comes to health. As we age, the body undergoes profound changes, making it crucial to adapt our lifestyle and diet to continue enjoying life to its fullest. For those diagnosed with diverticulitis or concerned about digestive health, embracing a tailored diet becomes not just a matter of choice but a vital aspect of everyday wellness.

This guide is designed with you in mind—offering not only recipes and meal plans but also the knowledge and support to manage and prevent flare-ups, ensuring that your digestive health doesn't hold you back from the joys of your senior years. This isn't just about avoiding certain foods; it's about discovering a new way to eat that enriches your body and life.

The journey through later life should be a delightful celebration of all you've achieved, and all that's yet to come, not marred by the pain and discomfort of digestive issues. Understanding the importance of dietary management as you age is the first step. As the digestive system ages, it becomes less efficient at processing certain types of food, making high-fiber diets increasingly important. Fiber helps to keep the digestive system flowing, reducing the pressure in the colon and, thus, the likelihood of flare-ups.

However, switching to a high-fiber diet is not merely about adding more bran to your morning cereal. It involves exploring a variety of nutrient-rich foods that not only delight the palate but also fortify the body against potential digestive troubles. For instance, integrating foods like oatmeal, raspberries, and flax seeds into your diet can significantly enhance your fiber intake without compromising on taste or variety.

Beyond individual ingredients, it's the method of preparation and the combination of foods that play an essential role in a diverticulitis-friendly diet. Cooking methods such as steaming, poaching, or baking over frying can preserve the integrity of the nutrients while making the food easier to digest. Complementing protein sources with fiber-rich sides ensures that each meal is balanced and promotes digestive health.

In these pages, you'll find recipes that cater specifically to the nutritional needs and taste preferences of seniors. From oatmeal with sliced pears and almond butter for a gentle start to the day to grilled salmon with dill and lemon for a fulfilling dinner, each recipe is crafted to provide maximum nutritional benefit without risking a flare-up. These meals are not only easy on the digestive system but are also crafted to be easy to prepare, recognizing that not every senior wants to spend long hours in the kitchen.

Moreover, adapting your diet as you age is about more than just what you eat—it's also about understanding how food interacts with your body and lifestyle. Factors like medication, mobility, and other health conditions can affect how your body processes food, which means dietary advice cannot be one-size-fits-all. This guide offers starting points and suggestions, but it is also flexible enough to be tailored to your specific needs and conditions. Personalization is key in managing health through diet, especially when dealing with a condition as variable as diverticulitis.

As part of this comprehensive approach, the book also dives into how lifestyle changes can support dietary adjustments. Regular, gentle exercise, adequate hydration, and stress management are all pivotal in maintaining digestive health and overall wellbeing. Techniques for managing stress, in particular, can have a profound impact on the frequency and severity of diverticulitis flare-ups. Mindfulness, meditation, and even simple breathing exercises can help manage stress levels and thus reduce the burden on your digestive system.

This guide is not only about managing a condition—it's about embracing a lifestyle that promotes digestive health and overall vitality. It's about making informed choices that enhance your quality of life, ensuring that your senior years are enjoyed with health, happiness, and peace of mind.

Remember, while aging is inevitable, suffering from chronic digestive issues doesn't have to be. With the right knowledge and tools, you can take proactive steps to manage your digestive health. This book is here to guide you through each step, offering practical advice, emotional support, and a community of peers and professionals who understand the challenges and rewards of managing diverticulitis in your golden years. Together, we can turn this phase of life into a vibrant journey of health and fulfillment.

CHAPTER 1

THE FOUNDATIONS OF A DIVERTICULITIS DIET

What is Diverticulitis?

Diverticulitis is a condition that emerges from diverticulosis, which involves the formation of small pouches, or diverticula, in the lining of the digestive tract. These pouches are most commonly found in the lower part of the large intestine (colon). While diverticulosis itself is generally symptom-free and harmless, complications arise when one or more of these pouches become inflamed or infected, leading to diverticulitis. This condition can cause significant discomfort and, depending on its severity, can severely impact a person's quality of life, especially for seniors.

Understanding the symptoms of diverticulitis is crucial for early detection and management. The most common symptom is abdominal pain, particularly in the lower left side of the abdomen, which can suddenly be severe. Other symptoms include fever, nausea, vomiting, chills, cramping, and constipation or, less commonly, diarrhea. The intensity of these symptoms can vary, with some episodes being mild and manageable at home, while others could be severe enough to require hospitalization.

For seniors, the impact of diverticulitis can be more pronounced. As we age, our bodies naturally become less resilient to illnesses and infections. The immune system weakens, making it harder to fight off infections, including those that can arise from diverticulitis. Additionally, the walls of the gastrointestinal tract thicken, and the muscles along the digestive pathway weaken, which can exacerbate the effects of diverticulitis. Seniors are more likely to experience complications such as perforations in the colon, abscesses, and blockages, which can be life-threatening if not treated promptly.

Moreover, many seniors are managing multiple health conditions simultaneously, which can complicate the treatment of diverticulitis. For instance, the medications used to manage other diseases might interact negatively with the antibiotics used to treat diverticulitis or may even worsen the condition itself. Anti-inflammatory drugs, commonly taken for conditions like arthritis, can increase the risk of bleeding in the presence of diverticulitis. Therefore, it's crucial for treatment plans to be personalized, taking into account the full spectrum of an individual's health profile.

Diet plays a pivotal role in both the management and prevention of diverticulitis, especially for seniors. A diet high in fiber can help keep the contents of the colon moving smoothly and reduce the pressure inside the digestive system, which can help prevent the formation of diverticula and decrease the chances of them becoming inflamed. However, during a flare-up of diverticulitis, a high-fiber diet could aggravate the condition, and a temporary shift to a low-fiber or liquid diet might be recommended to allow the colon to heal.

Adjusting to these dietary needs can be challenging, particularly for seniors who may have set eating habits or other dietary restrictions due to different health issues. It's essential for seniors and their caregivers to receive accurate dietary advice tailored to their specific needs, which can mitigate the risks associated with inappropriate diet management and ensure that nutrition remains balanced and beneficial.

Aside from diet, regular physical activity is encouraged as it helps maintain normal bowel function and reduces pressure inside the colon. However, the type and intensity of exercise should be appropriate for the senior's overall fitness level and mobility. Gentle activities like walking, swimming, or yoga can be beneficial without being overly strenuous.

Emotional and social support also play a critical role in managing diverticulitis, particularly for the elderly. The condition can be isolating, especially during severe flare-ups when individuals may not feel well enough to leave their homes. Support from family, friends, or support groups can provide not only practical help but also a psychological boost, helping seniors manage the stress and frustration that often comes with chronic conditions.

Understanding Diverticulitis After 60

As we age, the body undergoes significant physiological changes that can alter its response to various health conditions, including diverticulitis. These changes are particularly impactful after the age of 60, making it essential to understand how they can influence the course of the disease and the effectiveness of different treatment strategies, especially those related to diet.

One of the key changes in the body as we age is a decline in the strength and resilience of the digestive system. The walls of the gastrointestinal (GI) tract become thicker, and the muscles that facilitate digestion become weaker. This can slow down the transit time for food passing through the colon, which increases the risk of constipation—a common trigger for the development of diverticula and the onset of diverticulitis. The reduced motility of the colon not only predisposes older adults to the formation of diverticula but also increases the likelihood that these pouches will become inflamed or infected.

Additionally, the immune system's efficiency decreases with age, making it more challenging for the body to fight infections, including those in the GI tract. This reduced immune response can lead to a higher incidence of complications from diverticulitis in seniors, such as abscesses or perforations of the colon, which are serious conditions that require immediate medical attention.

Another age-related factor that influences the management of diverticulitis is the presence of comorbid conditions, such as diabetes, heart disease, or other digestive disorders like irritable bowel syndrome or inflammatory bowel disease. These conditions can complicate the management of diverticulitis because they might restrict the use of certain medications or necessitate specific dietary adjustments.

Given these complexities, targeted dietary strategies become crucial in managing diverticulitis in seniors. The traditional advice for managing diverticulitis has often centered on a high-fiber diet to help prevent constipation and minimize pressure in the colon. Fiber helps to soften stool and promotes quicker transit through the intestine, thus reducing the strain that can cause diverticula to form or become inflamed.

However, during a diverticulitis flare-up, a high-fiber diet can exacerbate symptoms. In such cases, medical professionals usually recommend a temporary shift to a low-fiber or clear liquid diet to allow the colon to heal. This dietary switch underscores the importance of personalized dietary planning for seniors with diverticulitis. It's essential to balance the long-term benefits of a high-fiber diet with the short-term needs of managing acute episodes of diverticulitis, all while considering the individual's overall health and other medical conditions.

Moreover, hydration plays a vital role in the management of diverticulitis. Adequate fluid intake helps fiber work better by helping to keep the stool soft and easier to pass. Seniors, however, often have a diminished sense of thirst, which can lead to insufficient fluid intake and dehydration, further complicating constipation and diverticulitis.

Nutritional considerations are also paramount. As digestion becomes less efficient with age, the body may not absorb nutrients as well from the diet. Seniors with diverticulitis need a well-rounded diet that provides all necessary nutrients without causing additional strain on the digestive system. This might include incorporating more easily digestible sources of fiber, such as cooked vegetables and fruits without skins and ensuring a sufficient intake of protein and essential fats.

Lastly, the role of a tailored diet extends beyond the physical aspects of managing diverticulitis. The diet also plays a significant role in a senior's quality of life, affecting their energy levels, mood, and overall sense of wellbeing. A diet that supports digestive health without causing discomfort can help seniors maintain an active and fulfilling lifestyle, even with diverticulitis.

Adapting Your Diet as You Age

As we move through the tapestry of our later years, the need to adapt our dietary habits becomes not only beneficial but essential. Aging changes the body in myriad ways, particularly how it processes and responds to food. For seniors, especially those managing conditions like diverticulitis, understanding how to modify eating habits is crucial for maintaining health and preventing painful flare-ups.

One of the most significant changes that occur as we age is the slowing down of the digestive system. This natural progression can lead to increased difficulties in digesting large meals and certain types of foods, notably those high in fat and low in fiber. Consequently, smaller, more frequent meals can be easier on an older digestive system, providing it with less to process at any given time and maintaining a steady flow through the digestive tract.

Fiber is particularly pivotal in an older adult's diet, given its role in enhancing digestion and preventing constipation, a common problem in later life that can exacerbate conditions like diverticulitis. A diet rich in fiber includes plenty of fruits, vegetables, whole grains, and legumes. These foods not only help keep the digestive system running smoothly but are also loaded with nutrients that are vital for maintaining overall health as we age.

However, it's not just about adding more fiber; it's about finding the right type of fiber. Soluble fiber, found in foods like oats, apples, and flaxseeds, dissolves in water to form a gel-like substance in the gut, helping to soften stool and support bowel health. Insoluble fiber, found in foods like whole grains and many vegetables, adds bulk to the stool and helps it pass more quickly and easily through the digestive system. Balancing these two types of fiber can help manage bowel health effectively.

Hydration also plays a crucial role in digestive health. Older adults often experience a reduced sense of thirst, which can lead to inadequate fluid intake and, subsequently, constipation. Drinking sufficient fluids, especially water can help manage and prevent digestive issues. Fluids also aid in the digestion and absorption of nutrients, making them a critical component of a senior's diet.

Adapting your diet as you age also means being mindful of how food interacts with medications. Many seniors take multiple medications, which can interact with certain foods and affect nutrient absorption. For instance, some medications may interfere with calcium absorption, making it important to find other ways to get this essential nutrient. Consulting with a healthcare provider or a nutritionist can help manage these interactions and ensure that the diet supports, rather than contradicts, medical treatments.

Reducing sodium intake is another dietary adaptation that is beneficial for seniors. High sodium consumption is linked to increased blood pressure, which poses significant health risks, such as heart disease and stroke. Instead of seasoning with salt, using herbs and spices can add flavor without the additional sodium, making meals enjoyable and healthier.

Equally important is the management of sugar intake. With age, the body's ability to regulate blood sugar levels can deteriorate, and high-sugar diets can lead to diabetes, among other health issues. Focusing on natural sugars found in fruits and balancing them with proteins and fats can help maintain energy levels and prevent blood sugar spikes.

Moreover, dietary needs vary widely among individuals, and what works for one senior may not work for another. Personalized diet plans that consider the individual's health conditions, dietary preferences, and nutritional needs are essential. This personalized approach ensures that dietary changes are not only effective in managing conditions like diverticulitis but are also sustainable and enjoyable, enhancing a senior's quality of life.

Adopting these dietary modifications can also foster a sense of control and empowerment—a feeling that is often diminished with age and health issues. Learning to adapt one's diet effectively can help seniors manage their health more proactively and maintain their independence.

How Aging Affects Digestive Health

As we age, our bodies undergo a multitude of changes, and the digestive system is no exception. These changes can significantly impact digestion, absorption, and overall gastrointestinal health. Understanding these physiological alterations and how to counteract their effects with dietary choices, particularly a high-fiber diet, is essential for maintaining health and quality of life in our later years.

The process of aging typically results in a reduction in the efficiency of the digestive system. One of the most noticeable changes is the slowing of gastrointestinal motility, which is the movement of food through the digestive tract. This slowdown can lead to a host of digestive problems, including an increased incidence of constipation, which is one of the most common gastrointestinal complaints among the elderly. The muscles in the digestive tract, including those in the esophagus, stomach, and intestines, become weaker and less efficient at pushing food through the system, causing delays in the digestion process and longer transit times.

In addition to slower motility, aging often brings a decrease in the production of digestive juices, such as stomach acid and digestive enzymes. This reduction can impair the body's ability to break down and absorb nutrients from food, particularly proteins, and certain vitamins and minerals, such as vitamin B12, calcium, and iron. The decreased absorption can lead to deficiencies, affecting overall health and exacerbating chronic conditions.

Another significant change is the alteration in the gut microbiota—the billions of bacteria that reside in the gastrointestinal tract. These bacteria play crucial roles in digestion, immune function, and even mood regulation. As we age, the diversity of these bacterial populations tends to decline, which can affect digestive health and increase susceptibility to infections such as Clostridioides difficile, a common cause of diarrhea in hospitalized elderly patients.

Given these challenges, incorporating a high-fiber diet becomes increasingly important as we age. Fiber plays several key roles in promoting healthy digestion and countering the effects of an aging digestive system. Firstly, fiber helps to increase stool bulk and softens it, making it easier to pass and reducing the risk of constipation. This is particularly beneficial given the slower gastrointestinal motility seen in the elderly.

Soluble fiber, found in foods like oats, apples, and beans, dissolves in water to form a gel-like substance in the gut. This gel helps regulate blood sugar levels by slowing the absorption of sugar, provides a feeling of fullness which can help with weight management, and can lower cholesterol levels by binding with cholesterol particles and removing them from the body. Insoluble fiber, found in whole grains, nuts, and vegetables, does not dissolve in water and adds bulk to the stool, which can help food pass more quickly through the stomach and intestines and ease the symptoms of a sluggish digestive tract.

Moreover, a high-fiber diet can also help nourish the gut microbiota. Many high-fiber foods are considered prebiotics, meaning they feed the good bacteria in the gut, promoting a healthy and diverse microbiota. This is crucial for elderly individuals whose microbiota may be diminished.

Despite the benefits, increasing fiber intake must be done cautiously for older adults. A sudden increase in fiber can lead to bloating, gas, or even constipation if not accompanied by adequate fluid intake. Therefore, it is important for seniors to increase their fiber intake gradually and ensure they are drinking plenty of fluids to help the fiber function properly in the digestive system.

In addition to dietary fiber, maintaining regular physical activity can also help improve gastrointestinal motility and support digestive health. Even gentle activities like walking can stimulate the muscles in the gastrointestinal tract and help facilitate smoother and more regular bowel movements.

The Connection Between Lifestyle and Digestive Flare-Ups

The interplay between lifestyle factors and digestive health is a subject of increasing interest and importance, particularly as it pertains to conditions such as diverticulitis. The onset and aggravation of diverticulitis flare-ups are significantly influenced by diet, exercise, and stress, making lifestyle management a cornerstone of effective treatment and prevention strategies.

Diet plays a pivotal role in the management of diverticulitis. Foods that are high in fiber, such as fruits, vegetables, and whole grains, are especially beneficial as they help maintain bowel regularity and prevent constipation, which can put undue pressure on the walls of the colon. This is crucial because increased pressure in the colon can lead to the formation of diverticula or exacerbate existing ones, thereby triggering diverticulitis episodes. A high-fiber diet not only helps in smoothing the passage of food through the digestive tract but also reduces the likelihood of the stool becoming too hard, which can irritate the diverticula.

Conversely, a diet rich in red meats, refined grains, and high-fat foods can increase the risk of diverticulitis flare-ups. These foods tend to be lower in fiber and higher in fats, which can slow down the digestive process, lead to overweight or obesity, and increase inflammation, all of which can worsen the symptoms of diverticulitis. Moreover, excessive consumption of alcohol and smoking has also been linked to an increased risk of developing diverticulitis, as they may cause inflammation of the diverticula and the intestinal lining.

Exercise is another lifestyle factor that greatly affects the frequency and severity of diverticulitis episodes. Regular physical activity helps stimulate the intestines, improving bowel motility and reducing the pressure inside the colon. This not only helps to prevent the formation of new diverticula but can also lessen the severity of the symptoms if a flare-up occurs. Furthermore, exercise is instrumental in maintaining a healthy weight, which is important because obesity is a known risk factor for diverticulitis. Obesity increases the strain on the colon and can make the abdominal cavity tighter, which might push against the diverticula and trigger inflammation.

Stress is equally significant in its impact on diverticulitis, though its effects are often underappreciated. Chronic stress can alter the gut flora and increase intestinal permeability, allowing bacteria to infiltrate the diverticula and cause infection. Stress also affects the rate of digestion; it can slow it down or speed it up, leading to diarrhea or constipation, both of which can exacerbate diverticulitis symptoms. Managing stress through techniques such as meditation, yoga, deep breathing exercises, or cognitive-behavioral strategies can therefore play a vital role in mitigating the frequency and severity of diverticulitis flare-ups.

Incorporating these lifestyle changes involves a holistic approach to health and wellbeing. Individuals suffering from diverticulitis should aim to adopt a balanced and nutritious diet that supports digestive health and enhances the immune system. This includes not only choosing the right foods but also preparing them in ways that preserve their nutritional content and are easy on the digestive system, such as steaming or baking instead of frying.

Regular, moderate exercise should be a part of the daily routine. Activities such as walking, cycling, or swimming are ideal because they stimulate the digestive system without being too strenuous. It's important for individuals to choose a form of exercise that they enjoy and can maintain regularly to ensure long-term adherence.

Stress management should also be prioritized. This might involve setting aside time for relaxation and leisure activities, seeking social support from friends and family, or even professional help if stress becomes overwhelming. Cultivating a positive mindset and learning to manage stress effectively can significantly improve the quality of life and reduce the impact of diverticulitis.

Key Dietary Principles to Follow

Diet plays a critical role in maintaining our health, particularly as we age and our bodies require more careful management to prevent and manage conditions such as diverticulitis. The guidelines laid out in this book are designed to provide a foundation for a diet that supports not just the digestive system but overall wellbeing. By adhering to these core principles, individuals can enhance their quality of life, mitigate the risks associated with digestive disorders, and enjoy their later years with vitality and pleasure.

The first principle revolves around the importance of a high-fiber diet. Fiber is paramount for maintaining smooth and regular bowel movements, which is crucial in preventing the strain and pressure that can lead to the formation and exacerbation of diverticula. Sources of fiber such as fruits, vegetables, legumes, and whole grains should be incorporated into daily meals in ample quantities. These foods not only aid in digestion but also provide a host of other nutrients that are beneficial for health. It is important, however, to increase fiber intake gradually to allow the body to adjust without causing discomfort such as bloating or gas.

Hydration is another key aspect of the dietary guidelines. Water plays an essential role in digestion by helping to dissolve nutrients and fiber, facilitating their movement through the digestive system, and aiding in the efficient absorption of nutrients. Drinking sufficient water throughout the day can prevent dehydration, which is a common issue among seniors and a frequent cause of constipation. It can also reduce the risk of diverticulitis flare-ups by ensuring that waste moves through the colon more easily.

Protein intake must also be carefully managed. As we age, maintaining muscle mass becomes more challenging, making adequate protein intake essential. However, choosing the right types of protein is crucial. Lean proteins such as chicken, turkey, and fish, as well as plant-based proteins like beans and lentils, are preferable. These foods provide the necessary nutrients without excessive fats that can exacerbate digestive problems. Reducing the intake of red and processed meats, which have been linked to an increased risk of diverticulitis and other health issues, is also recommended.

Reducing the intake of refined sugars and fats is crucial for digestive health. Foods high in refined sugars can alter the balance of gut bacteria and exacerbate inflammation, while excessive fatty foods can slow down the digestive process, leading to a higher risk of constipation and diverticulitis flare-ups. Instead, focus on consuming natural sugars from fruits and healthier fats from sources like avocados, nuts, seeds, and olive oil. These changes can help maintain energy levels, support immune function, and ensure that the digestive system operates smoothly.

Another important guideline is the moderation of dairy products. For those who tolerate dairy well, products like yogurt and kefir can provide beneficial probiotics that support gut health. However, for those who are lactose intolerant or find dairy products to exacerbate their symptoms, alternatives such as lactose-free milk or plant-based milk enriched with calcium can be excellent substitutes.

The dietary guidelines also emphasize the importance of meal timing and portion control. Eating smaller, more frequent meals can prevent the digestive system from becoming overloaded, a common problem that can lead to discomfort and increased pressure in the colon. This approach not only aids in digestion but can also help regulate blood sugar levels and manage appetite more effectively.

Managing alcohol and caffeine consumption is also advisable. Both substances can irritate the digestive tract and should be consumed in moderation. For those with diverticulitis, particularly during flare-ups, avoiding alcohol and caffeine can prevent aggravation of symptoms and promote healing.

Lastly, the role of antioxidants and anti-inflammatory foods cannot be overstated. Foods rich in antioxidants, such as berries, nuts, and green leafy vegetables, can help combat oxidative stress, which increases with age and can exacerbate many chronic health conditions, including diverticulitis. Similarly, incorporating anti-inflammatory foods like turmeric, ginger, and fatty fish can help reduce inflammation in the body, including the digestive system.

Incorporating these dietary guidelines into daily life requires commitment and gradual change. It is about making informed choices that not only aim to prevent flare-ups of diverticulitis but also contribute to a more energetic and fulfilling lifestyle. These changes can help ensure that dietary management of diverticulitis is not about restriction but about enhancing life through better health practices. As each individual is unique, it is important to tailor these guidelines to personal health conditions, preferences, and nutritional needs, ideally under the guidance of healthcare professionals. This personalized approach will ensure that the diet not only prevents digestive issues but also supports a vibrant, healthy life in the golden years.

Thank you for beginning this journey with us through "Diverticulitis Diet After 60." We hope the information in the first chapter has provided valuable insights into managing your dietary needs effectively. Your feedback is crucial to us as it helps us understand your experiences and improve our guidance.

How You Can Share Your Review:

Through Amazon.com:

- Go to the Amazon page where you found my book.

- Navigate to the 'Customer Reviews' section.

- Click on 'Write a customer review' to share your valuable insights.

Instant QR Code Access: Simply scan the QR code below with your smartphone to be directed to the Amazon review section.

CHAPTER 2

BREAKFAST RECIPES

Oatmeal with Sliced Pears and Almond Butter

Ingredients:

- 1/2 cup rolled oats
- 1 cup water or milk (or a mix of both)
- 1 medium pear, thinly sliced
- 1 tablespoon almond butter
- 1/4 teaspoon cinnamon
- Optional: 1 teaspoon honey or maple syrup for sweetness

Directions:

1. In a small saucepan, bring water or milk to a boil.
2. Stir in the rolled oats and reduce the heat to a simmer. Cook for about 5 minutes, stirring occasionally, until the oats are soft and the liquid is absorbed.
3. While the oats are cooking, prepare the pear by slicing it thinly.
4. Once the oatmeal is ready, remove it from the heat and stir in the cinnamon.
5. Transfer the oatmeal to a bowl and top it with the sliced pears.
6. Drizzle the almond butter over the top. If desired, add honey or maple syrup for extra sweetness.
7. Serve warm.

Nutritional Values:

- Calories: 300
- Fat: 10g
- Carbohydrates: 48g
- Protein: 7g

Buckwheat Pancakes with Blueberry Compote

Ingredients:

- 1 cup buckwheat flour
- 1 tablespoon sugar
- 1 teaspoon baking powder
- 1/4 teaspoon salt

- 1 cup milk (dairy or non-dairy)

- 1 large egg

- 2 tablespoons melted butter or oil

- 1 cup fresh or frozen blueberries

- 2 tablespoons maple syrup

Directions:

1. In a large bowl, whisk together the buckwheat flour, sugar, baking powder, and salt.

2. In another bowl, whisk the milk, egg, and melted butter or oil until well combined.

3. Pour the wet ingredients into the dry ingredients and stir until just combined; the batter should be slightly lumpy.

4. Heat a non-stick skillet over medium heat and lightly grease it. Pour 1/4 cup of batter onto the skillet for each pancake.

5. Cook until bubbles form on the surface, then flip and cook the other side until golden brown, about 2-3 minutes per side.

6. For the compote, heat the blueberries and maple syrup in a small saucepan over medium heat until the blueberries burst and the mixture thickens slightly.

7. Serve the pancakes topped with warm blueberry compote.

Nutritional Values:

- Calories: 350

- Fat: 12g

- Carbohydrates: 52g

- Protein: 10g

Scrambled Eggs with Spinach and Mushrooms

Ingredients:

- 3 large eggs

- 1/4 cup milk

- 1 cup fresh spinach leaves

- 1/2 cup sliced mushrooms

- 1 tablespoon olive oil or butter

- Salt and pepper to taste

Directions:

1. In a bowl, whisk the eggs and milk together until well combined. Season with salt and pepper.

2. Heat the olive oil or butter in a non-stick skillet over medium heat. Add the mushrooms and cook until they are soft and browned, about 4-5 minutes.

3. Add the spinach to the skillet and cook until wilted, about 1-2 minutes.

4. Pour the egg mixture over the vegetables in the skillet. Stir gently and continuously until the eggs are

fully cooked and scrambled, about 3-4 minutes.

5. Serve immediately.

Nutritional Values:

- Calories: 250
- Fat: 18g
- Carbohydrates: 5g
- Protein: 18g

Quinoa Porridge with Apple and Cinnamon

Ingredients:

- 1/2 cup quinoa, rinsed
- 1 cup water or milk (or a mix of both)
- 1 small apple, chopped
- 1/4 teaspoon cinnamon
- 1 tablespoon honey or maple syrup
- Optional: nuts or seeds for topping

Directions:

1. In a medium saucepan, bring the water or milk to a boil. Add the rinsed quinoa, reduce heat to low, and cover. Cook for about 15 minutes, or until the quinoa is tender and the liquid is absorbed.

2. While the quinoa is cooking, sauté the chopped apple in a small pan over medium heat with a sprinkle of cinnamon until soft.

3. Once the quinoa is cooked, stir in the cinnamon and honey or maple syrup.

4. Serve the quinoa porridge in a bowl topped with the sautéed apples and any optional toppings like nuts or seeds.

Nutritional Values:

- Calories: 300
- Fat: 6g
- Carbohydrates: 55g
- Protein: 8g

Smoothie Bowl with Banana, Kiwi, and Flaxseed

Ingredients:

- 1 banana, sliced and frozen
- 1/2 cup plain Greek yogurt
- 1/4 cup milk (dairy or non-dairy)
- 1 kiwi, peeled and sliced
- 1 tablespoon flaxseed
- Optional: granola, nuts, or seeds for topping

Directions:

1. In a blender, combine the frozen banana, Greek yogurt, and milk. Blend until smooth and thick.

2. Pour the smoothie into a bowl.

3. Top with sliced kiwi and sprinkle with flaxseed.

4. Add any additional toppings like granola, nuts, or seeds as desired.

5. Serve immediately.

Nutritional Values:

- Calories: 300
- Fat: 10g
- Carbohydrates: 45g
- Protein: 12g

Chia Pudding with Coconut Milk and Mango

Ingredients:

- 1/4 cup chia seeds
- 1 cup coconut milk
- 1 tablespoon honey or maple syrup
- 1/2 cup diced mango

Directions:

1. In a bowl, whisk together the chia seeds, coconut milk, and honey or maple syrup.

2. Cover and refrigerate for at least 4 hours or overnight, until the mixture has thickened into a pudding-like consistency.

3. Stir the chia pudding and divide it into serving bowls.

4. Top with diced mango and serve chilled.

Nutritional Values:

- Calories: 350
- Fat: 22g
- Carbohydrates: 32g
- Protein: 5g

Barley Breakfast Salad with Citrus and Walnuts

Ingredients:

- 1/2 cup cooked barley
- 1 orange, segmented
- 1/4 cup chopped walnuts
- 1 tablespoon olive oil
- 1 tablespoon lemon juice
- Salt and pepper to taste

Directions:

1. In a bowl, combine the cooked barley, orange segments, and chopped walnuts.

2. In a small bowl, whisk together the olive oil and lemon juice. Pour over the barley mixture.

3. Toss gently to combine and season with salt and pepper.

4. Serve at room temperature or chilled.

Nutritional Values:

- Calories: 300
- Fat: 15g
- Carbohydrates: 40g
- Protein: 6g

Whole Wheat Toast with Avocado and Poached Egg

Ingredients:

- 1 slice whole wheat bread, toasted
- 1/2 avocado, mashed
- 1 large egg
- 1 tablespoon vinegar (for poaching)
- Salt and pepper to taste
- Optional: red pepper flakes or herbs for topping

Directions:

1. Bring a pot of water to a gentle simmer and add the vinegar.
2. Crack the egg into a small bowl and gently slide it into the simmering water. Poach the egg for 3-4 minutes, or until the white is set but the yolk is still runny.
3. While the egg is poaching, spread the mashed avocado on the toasted bread.
4. Carefully remove the poached egg with a slotted spoon and place it on top of the avocado toast.
5. Season with salt, pepper, and any optional toppings.
6. Serve immediately.

Nutritional Values:

- Calories: 250
- Fat: 18g
- Carbohydrates: 20g
- Protein: 8g

Baked Sweet Potato and Kale Hash

Ingredients:

- 1 large sweet potato, peeled and diced
- 1 cup kale, chopped
- 1/2 onion, diced
- 1 tablespoon olive oil
- Salt and pepper to taste
- Optional: 1/4 teaspoon smoked paprika

Directions:

1. Preheat the oven to 400°F (200°C).
2. Toss the diced sweet potato, kale, and onion with olive oil, salt, pepper, and smoked paprika if using.
3. Spread the mixture evenly on a baking sheet.

4. Bake for 20-25 minutes, or until the sweet potatoes are tender and slightly crisp.

5. Serve hot as a side dish or a main course.

Nutritional Values:

- Calories: 220
- Fat: 8g
- Carbohydrates: 35g
- Protein: 4g

Millet Cereal with Raisins and Honey

Ingredients:

- 1/2 cup millet
- 1 cup water or milk (or a mix of both)
- 1/4 cup raisins
- 1 tablespoon honey
- Optional: a pinch of cinnamon or nutmeg

Directions:

1. In a small saucepan, bring water or milk to a boil.

2. Add the millet, reduce the heat, and simmer for about 20 minutes, or until the millet is tender and the liquid is absorbed.

3. Stir in the raisins, honey, and optional spices.

4. Serve warm, with additional milk or honey if desired.

Nutritional Values:

- Calories: 300
- Fat: 4g
- Carbohydrates: 60g
- Protein: 6g

Rice Cakes Topped with Ricotta and Fresh Berries

Ingredients:

- 2 rice cakes
- 1/4 cup ricotta cheese
- 1/2 cup fresh berries (strawberries, blueberries, or raspberries)
- Optional: a drizzle of honey or maple syrup

Directions:

1. Spread the ricotta cheese evenly over the rice cakes.

2. Top with fresh berries.

3. Drizzle with honey or maple syrup if desired.

4. Serve immediately.

Nutritional Values:

- Calories: 180
- Fat: 6g
- Carbohydrates: 28g

- Protein: 5g

Sautéed Tofu with Asparagus and Tomatoes

Ingredients:

- 1/2 block firm tofu, drained and cubed
- 1 cup asparagus, chopped
- 1/2 cup cherry tomatoes, halved
- 1 tablespoon olive oil
- 1 clove garlic, minced
- Salt and pepper to taste

Directions:

1. Heat the olive oil in a skillet over medium heat. Add the garlic and sauté until fragrant, about 1 minute.
2. Add the tofu cubes to the skillet and cook until golden brown on all sides, about 5-7 minutes.
3. Add the asparagus and cook for another 3-4 minutes, until tender.
4. Stir in the cherry tomatoes and cook for an additional 2 minutes.
5. Season with salt and pepper, and serve hot.

Nutritional Values:

- Calories: 250
- Fat: 15g
- Carbohydrates: 10g

- Protein: 18g

Multigrain Waffles with Strawberry Sauce

Ingredients:

- 1 cup multigrain flour
- 1 tablespoon sugar
- 1 teaspoon baking powder
- 1/4 teaspoon salt
- 1 cup milk (dairy or non-dairy)
- 1 large egg
- 2 tablespoons melted butter or oil
- 1 cup fresh strawberries, sliced
- 2 tablespoons maple syrup

Directions:

1. In a large bowl, whisk together the multigrain flour, sugar, baking powder, and salt.
2. In another bowl, whisk the milk, egg, and melted butter or oil until well combined.
3. Pour the wet ingredients into the dry ingredients and stir until just combined; the batter should be slightly lumpy.
4. Preheat a waffle iron and lightly grease it.
5. Pour the batter into the waffle iron and cook according to the

manufacturer's instructions until golden brown.

6. Meanwhile, heat the strawberries and maple syrup in a small saucepan until the strawberries soften and release their juices.

7. Serve the waffles topped with warm strawberry sauce.

Nutritional Values:

- Calories: 350

- Fat: 12g

- Carbohydrates: 52g

- Protein: 10g

Savory Oatmeal with Grated Zucchini and Thyme

Ingredients:

- 1/2 cup rolled oats

- 1 cup water or broth

- 1/2 small zucchini, grated

- 1/4 teaspoon fresh thyme leaves

- 1 tablespoon grated Parmesan cheese

- Salt and pepper to taste

Directions:

1. In a small saucepan, bring water or broth to a boil.

2. Stir in the rolled oats and reduce the heat to a simmer. Cook for about 5 minutes, stirring occasionally.

3. Stir in the grated zucchini and thyme and cook for another 2 minutes.

4. Remove from heat and stir in the Parmesan cheese.

5. Season with salt and pepper, and serve warm.

Nutritional Values:

- Calories: 220

- Fat: 6g

- Carbohydrates: 35g

- Protein: 8g

Cottage Cheese with Sliced Peaches and Pumpkin Seeds

Ingredients:

- 1/2 cup cottage cheese

- 1 small peach, sliced

- 1 tablespoon pumpkin seeds

- Optional: a drizzle of honey or cinnamon

Directions:

1. Spoon the cottage cheese into a serving bowl.

2. Top with sliced peaches and pumpkin seeds.

3. Drizzle with honey or sprinkle with cinnamon if desired.

4. Serve immediately.

Nutritional Values:

- Calories: 180
- Fat: 6g
- Carbohydrates: 15g
- Protein: 14g

Greek Yogurt with Homemade Granola and Apple Slices

Ingredients:

- 1 cup Greek yogurt (plain, unsweetened)
- 1/4 cup homemade granola
- 1 small apple, thinly sliced
- Optional: a drizzle of honey or maple syrup

Directions:

1. Spoon the Greek yogurt into a serving bowl.

2. Top with granola and apple slices.

3. Drizzle with honey or maple syrup if desired.

4. Serve immediately.

Nutritional Values:

- Calories: 250

- Fat: 8g
- Carbohydrates: 32g
- Protein: 15g

Soft-Boiled Egg with Asparagus Soldiers

Ingredients:

- 1 large egg
- 5-6 asparagus spears, trimmed
- 1 teaspoon olive oil
- Salt and pepper to taste

Directions:

1. Bring a small pot of water to a boil. Gently lower the egg into the water and cook for 5-6 minutes for a soft-boiled egg.

2. While the egg is cooking, toss the asparagus spears with olive oil, salt, and pepper.

3. Grill or sauté the asparagus until tender, about 3-4 minutes.

4. Remove the egg from the boiling water and place it in an egg cup. Crack the top and serve with asparagus spears for dipping.

5. Serve immediately.

Nutritional Values:

- Calories: 150
- Fat: 10g

- Carbohydrates: 4g
- Protein: 10g

Breakfast Lentils with Carrots and Celery

Ingredients:

- 1/2 cup lentils, rinsed
- 1 cup water or broth
- 1 small carrot, diced
- 1 celery stalk, diced
- 1 tablespoon olive oil
- Salt and pepper to taste

Directions:

1. In a saucepan, bring the lentils and water or broth to a boil. Reduce the heat and simmer for about 20 minutes, until the lentils are tender.
2. Meanwhile, sauté the carrot and celery in olive oil until softened, about 5 minutes.
3. Stir the sautéed vegetables into the cooked lentils and season with salt and pepper.
4. Serve warm.

Nutritional Values:

- Calories: 220
- Fat: 8g
- Carbohydrates: 30g
- Protein: 10g

Spelt Muffins with Pear and Ginger

Ingredients:

- 1 1/2 cups spelt flour
- 1 teaspoon baking powder
- 1/4 teaspoon salt
- 1/2 teaspoon ground ginger
- 1/2 cup honey or maple syrup
- 1/4 cup melted butter or oil
- 1 large egg
- 1 cup diced pear

Directions:

1. Preheat the oven to 350°F (175°C) and line a muffin tin with paper liners.
2. In a large bowl, whisk together the spelt flour, baking powder, salt, and ground ginger.
3. In another bowl, whisk together the honey or maple syrup, melted butter or oil, and egg.
4. Pour the wet ingredients into the dry ingredients and stir until just combined.
5. Fold in the diced pear.
6. Divide the batter evenly among the muffin cups.

7. Bake for 20-25 minutes, or until a toothpick inserted into the center comes out clean.

8. Cool on a wire rack before serving.

Nutritional Values:

- Calories: 180 per muffin

- Fat: 6g

- Carbohydrates: 30g

- Protein: 4g

Polenta with Roasted Tomatoes and Basil

Ingredients:

- 1/2 cup polenta

- 1 1/2 cups water or broth

- 1/4 cup grated Parmesan cheese

- 1 cup cherry tomatoes, halved

- 1 tablespoon olive oil

- 1/4 cup fresh basil leaves, chopped

- Salt and pepper to taste

Directions:

1. Preheat the oven to 400°F (200°C).

2. Toss the cherry tomatoes with olive oil, salt, and pepper, and spread them on a baking sheet. Roast for 15-20 minutes, until softened and slightly caramelized.

3. Meanwhile, bring water or broth to a boil in a saucepan. Gradually whisk in the polenta, reduce the heat, and simmer, stirring constantly, until thickened, about 5 minutes.

4. Stir in the grated Parmesan cheese and season with salt and pepper.

5. Serve the polenta topped with roasted tomatoes and fresh basil.

Nutritional Values:

- Calories: 250

- Fat: 10g

- Carbohydrates: 32g

- Protein: 7g

CHAPTER 3

LUNCH RECIPES

Lentil Soup with Carrots and Celery

Ingredients:

- 1 cup dried lentils, rinsed
- 1 tablespoon olive oil
- 1 onion, diced
- 2 carrots, diced
- 2 celery stalks, diced
- 3 garlic cloves, minced
- 1 teaspoon ground cumin
- 1/2 teaspoon dried thyme
- 6 cups vegetable broth
- Salt and pepper to taste
- Optional: fresh parsley for garnish

Directions:

1. In a large pot, heat olive oil over medium heat. Add the onion, carrots, and celery, and cook until softened, about 5 minutes.
2. Stir in the garlic, cumin, and thyme, and cook for another minute until fragrant.
3. Add the lentils and vegetable broth, and bring to a boil.
4. Reduce the heat and simmer for 25-30 minutes, or until the lentils are tender.
5. Season with salt and pepper, and garnish with fresh parsley if desired.
6. Serve hot.

Nutritional Values:

- Calories: 250
- Fat: 5g
- Carbohydrates: 40g
- Protein: 12g

Quinoa Tabbouleh with Cucumbers and Mint

Ingredients:

- 1 cup cooked quinoa
- 1 cucumber, diced

* 1 cup cherry tomatoes, halved
* 1/4 cup fresh mint leaves, chopped
* 1/4 cup fresh parsley, chopped
* 2 tablespoons olive oil
* 2 tablespoons lemon juice
* Salt and pepper to taste

Directions:

1. In a large bowl, combine the cooked quinoa, diced cucumber, cherry tomatoes, mint, and parsley.

2. In a small bowl, whisk together the olive oil and lemon juice.

3. Pour the dressing over the quinoa mixture and toss to combine.

4. Season with salt and pepper to taste.

5. Serve chilled or at room temperature.

Nutritional Values:

* Calories: 220
* Fat: 10g
* Carbohydrates: 28g
* Protein: 6g

Baked Salmon with Dill and Lemon

Ingredients:

* 2 salmon fillets
* 1 tablespoon olive oil
* 1 lemon, sliced
* 1 tablespoon fresh dill, chopped
* Salt and pepper to taste

Directions:

1. Preheat the oven to 400°F (200°C).

2. Place the salmon fillets on a baking sheet lined with parchment paper.

3. Drizzle the salmon with olive oil and season with salt and pepper.

4. Top each fillet with lemon slices and sprinkle with fresh dill.

5. Bake for 12-15 minutes, or until the salmon is cooked through and flakes easily with a fork.

6. Serve immediately.

Nutritional Values:

* Calories: 300
* Fat: 20g
* Carbohydrates: 2g
* Protein: 25g

Grilled Chicken Salad with Mixed Greens and Avocado

Ingredients:

* 1 chicken breast, grilled and sliced
* 4 cups mixed salad greens
* 1 avocado, sliced
* 1/2 cup cherry tomatoes, halved

- 1/4 cup red onion, thinly sliced

- 2 tablespoons olive oil

- 1 tablespoon balsamic vinegar

- Salt and pepper to taste

Directions:

1. In a large salad bowl, combine the mixed greens, avocado, cherry tomatoes, and red onion.

2. Top with the grilled chicken slices.

3. In a small bowl, whisk together the olive oil and balsamic vinegar.

4. Drizzle the dressing over the salad and toss to combine.

5. Season with salt and pepper to taste.

6. Serve immediately.

Nutritional Values:

- Calories: 350

- Fat: 25g

- Carbohydrates: 10g

- Protein: 22g

Vegetable Stir-Fry with Tofu and Tamari Sauce

Ingredients:

- 1/2 block firm tofu, cubed

- 1 tablespoon olive oil

- 1 bell pepper, sliced

- 1 zucchini, sliced

- 1 carrot, julienned

- 1 cup broccoli florets

- 2 tablespoons tamari sauce (or soy sauce)

- 1 tablespoon sesame seeds

- Optional: 1 teaspoon grated ginger

Directions:

1. Heat olive oil in a large skillet over medium heat. Add the tofu cubes and cook until golden brown on all sides, about 5-7 minutes.

2. Remove the tofu and set aside. Add the bell pepper, zucchini, carrot, and broccoli to the skillet. Stir-fry for 5-7 minutes, until the vegetables are tender but still crisp.

3. Return the tofu to the skillet and pour in the tamari sauce. Stir to combine and cook for another 2 minutes.

4. Sprinkle with sesame seeds and serve hot.

Nutritional Values:

- Calories: 280

- Fat: 15g

- Carbohydrates: 20g

- Protein: 15g

Turkey and Spinach Wrap with Whole Wheat Tortilla

Ingredients:

- 1 whole wheat tortilla
- 2-3 slices turkey breast
- 1/2 cup fresh spinach leaves
- 1/4 cup shredded carrots
- 1 tablespoon hummus or mustard
- Salt and pepper to taste

Directions:

1. Lay the whole wheat tortilla flat on a plate.
2. Spread hummus or mustard evenly over the tortilla.
3. Layer the turkey slices, spinach leaves, and shredded carrots on top.
4. Season with salt and pepper if desired.
5. Roll up the tortilla tightly and slice in half.
6. Serve immediately.

Nutritional Values:

- Calories: 250
- Fat: 7g
- Carbohydrates: 30g
- Protein: 15g

Beetroot and Goat Cheese Arugula Salad

Ingredients:

- 2 medium beetroots, roasted and sliced
- 4 cups arugula
- 1/4 cup crumbled goat cheese
- 2 tablespoons olive oil
- 1 tablespoon balsamic vinegar
- Salt and pepper to taste

Directions:

1. In a large salad bowl, combine the arugula and roasted beetroot slices.
2. Sprinkle the crumbled goat cheese over the top.
3. In a small bowl, whisk together the olive oil and balsamic vinegar.
4. Drizzle the dressing over the salad and toss to combine.
5. Season with salt and pepper to taste.
6. Serve immediately.

Nutritional Values:

- Calories: 220
- Fat: 14g
- Carbohydrates: 18g
- Protein: 6g

Stuffed Bell Peppers with Brown Rice and Herbs

Ingredients:

- 4 bell peppers, tops cut off and seeds removed
- 1 cup cooked brown rice
- 1/2 onion, diced
- 1/2 cup diced tomatoes
- 1/4 cup fresh parsley, chopped
- 1 tablespoon olive oil
- Salt and pepper to taste

Directions:

1. Preheat the oven to 375°F (190°C).
2. In a large bowl, combine the cooked brown rice, diced onion, tomatoes, parsley, olive oil, salt, and pepper.
3. Stuff each bell pepper with the rice mixture and place in a baking dish.
4. Cover the dish with foil and bake for 30-35 minutes, or until the peppers are tender.
5. Serve hot.

Nutritional Values:

- Calories: 250
- Fat: 8g
- Carbohydrates: 40g
- Protein: 5g

Butternut Squash Soup with a Hint of Ginger

Ingredients:

- 1 medium butternut squash, peeled and cubed
- 1 onion, diced
- 1 tablespoon olive oil
- 1 teaspoon grated fresh ginger
- 4 cups vegetable broth
- Salt and pepper to taste
- Optional: a dollop of Greek yogurt for garnish

Directions:

1. In a large pot, heat olive oil over medium heat. Add the onion and ginger, and cook until the onion is soft, about 5 minutes.
2. Add the cubed butternut squash and vegetable broth. Bring to a boil, then reduce heat and simmer for 20-25 minutes, until the squash is tender.
3. Use an immersion blender to puree the soup until smooth. Alternatively, transfer the soup to a blender and blend in batches.
4. Season with salt and pepper to taste.
5. Serve hot, with a dollop of Greek yogurt if desired.

Nutritional Values:

- Calories: 180
- Fat: 5g
- Carbohydrates: 32g
- Protein: 4g

Pan-Seared Cod with Fennel and Orange Salad

Ingredients:

- 2 cod fillets
- 1 tablespoon olive oil
- 1 bulb fennel, thinly sliced
- 1 orange, segmented
- 1 tablespoon fresh lemon juice
- Salt and pepper to taste

Directions:

1. Heat olive oil in a large skillet over medium heat. Season the cod fillets with salt and pepper.

2. Place the fillets in the skillet and cook for 3-4 minutes per side, or until the fish is cooked through and flakes easily with a fork.

3. In a large bowl, combine the fennel slices, orange segments, and lemon juice.

4. Toss to combine and season with salt and pepper.

5. Serve the cod fillets with the fennel and orange salad on the side.

Nutritional Values:

- Calories: 250
- Fat: 10g
- Carbohydrates: 15g
- Protein: 28g

Mediterranean Chickpea and Eggplant Stew

Ingredients:

- 1 eggplant, diced
- 1 can chickpeas, drained and rinsed
- 1 can diced tomatoes
- 1 onion, diced
- 2 garlic cloves, minced
- 1 tablespoon olive oil
- 1 teaspoon ground cumin
- 1/2 teaspoon smoked paprika
- Salt and pepper to taste

Directions:

1. Heat olive oil in a large pot over medium heat. Add the onion and garlic, and cook until softened, about 5 minutes.

2. Add the diced eggplant, cumin, and smoked paprika, and cook for another 5 minutes.

3. Stir in the chickpeas and diced tomatoes. Bring to a boil, then

reduce heat and simmer for 20-25 minutes, until the eggplant is tender.

4. Season with salt and pepper to taste.

5. Serve hot, optionally garnished with fresh herbs.

Nutritional Values:

- Calories: 300

- Fat: 10g

- Carbohydrates: 40g

- Protein: 8g

Cauliflower Rice with Grilled Zucchini and Pesto

Ingredients:

- 1 head cauliflower, grated into rice-sized pieces

- 1 zucchini, sliced

- 2 tablespoons olive oil

- 2 tablespoons pesto

- Salt and pepper to taste

Directions:

1. Heat 1 tablespoon of olive oil in a large skillet over medium heat. Add the grated cauliflower and cook for 5-7 minutes, until tender.

2. In a separate pan, heat the remaining olive oil and grill the zucchini slices until tender and slightly charred, about 3-4 minutes per side.

3. Toss the cooked cauliflower rice with the pesto and season with salt and pepper.

4. Serve the cauliflower rice topped with the grilled zucchini slices.

Nutritional Values:

- Calories: 200

- Fat: 15g

- Carbohydrates: 10g

- Protein: 4g

Vegetable Paella with Saffron and Artichokes

Ingredients:

- 1 cup arborio rice

- 1 onion, diced

- 1 red bell pepper, diced

- 1 cup artichoke hearts, quartered

- 2 garlic cloves, minced

- 1 tablespoon olive oil

- 1/4 teaspoon saffron threads

- 4 cups vegetable broth

- 1/2 cup peas

- Salt and pepper to taste

Directions:

1. Heat olive oil in a large skillet over medium heat. Add the onion, bell

pepper, and garlic, and cook until softened, about 5 minutes.

2. Stir in the arborio rice and saffron, and cook for another 2 minutes, until the rice is lightly toasted.

3. Add the vegetable broth and bring to a boil. Reduce heat to low, cover, and simmer for 15 minutes.

4. Stir in the artichoke hearts and peas, and continue to cook for another 10 minutes, until the rice is tender and the liquid is absorbed.

5. Season with salt and pepper to taste, and serve hot.

Nutritional Values:

- Calories: 300
- Fat: 8g
- Carbohydrates: 55g
- Protein: 7g

Broccoli and Purple Cabbage Coleslaw

Ingredients:

- 1 cup shredded broccoli
- 1 cup shredded purple cabbage
- 1 carrot, grated
- 2 tablespoons Greek yogurt
- 1 tablespoon apple cider vinegar
- 1 tablespoon honey
- Salt and pepper to taste

Directions:

1. In a large bowl, combine the shredded broccoli, cabbage, and grated carrot.

2. In a small bowl, whisk together the Greek yogurt, apple cider vinegar, and honey.

3. Pour the dressing over the vegetable mixture and toss to combine.

4. Season with salt and pepper to taste.

5. Serve chilled.

Nutritional Values:

- Calories: 150
- Fat: 4g
- Carbohydrates: 25g
- Protein: 5g

Sweet Potato and Black Bean Burrito

Ingredients:

- 1 large sweet potato, peeled and diced
- 1 can black beans, drained and rinsed
- 1/2 cup corn kernels
- 1 tablespoon olive oil
- 1/2 teaspoon cumin
- 1/4 teaspoon chili powder

- Salt and pepper to taste

- 2 whole wheat tortillas

- Optional: avocado, salsa, or cheese for topping

Directions:

1. Preheat the oven to 400°F (200°C).

2. Toss the diced sweet potato with olive oil, cumin, chili powder, salt, and pepper. Spread on a baking sheet and roast for 20-25 minutes, until tender.

3. In a large bowl, combine the roasted sweet potatoes, black beans, and corn.

4. Warm the tortillas in a dry skillet or microwave.

5. Divide the sweet potato mixture between the tortillas and wrap them up.

6. Serve with optional toppings like avocado, salsa, or cheese.

Nutritional Values:

- Calories: 350

- Fat: 10g

- Carbohydrates: 60g

- Protein: 10g

Tomato and Basil Bruschetta on Whole Grain Bread

Ingredients:

- 4 slices whole grain bread, toasted

- 2 large tomatoes, diced

- 1/4 cup fresh basil, chopped

- 1 garlic clove, minced

- 2 tablespoons olive oil

- Salt and pepper to taste

Directions:

1. In a medium bowl, combine the diced tomatoes, basil, garlic, and olive oil.

2. Season with salt and pepper to taste.

3. Spoon the tomato mixture onto the toasted whole grain bread slices.

4. Serve immediately.

Nutritional Values:

- Calories: 200

- Fat: 10g

- Carbohydrates: 24g

- Protein: 4g

Spicy Pumpkin Soup with Coconut Milk

Ingredients:

- 1 can pumpkin puree

- 1 onion, diced

- 1 tablespoon olive oil

- 1 teaspoon ground cumin

- 1/4 teaspoon cayenne pepper

- 1 can coconut milk

- 2 cups vegetable broth

- Salt and pepper to taste

Directions:

1. In a large pot, heat olive oil over medium heat. Add the onion, cumin, and cayenne pepper, and cook until the onion is soft, about 5 minutes.

2. Stir in the pumpkin puree, coconut milk, and vegetable broth. Bring to a boil, then reduce heat and simmer for 15-20 minutes.

3. Use an immersion blender to puree the soup until smooth. Alternatively, transfer the soup to a blender and blend in batches.

4. Season with salt and pepper to taste.

5. Serve hot.

Nutritional Values:

- Calories: 300

- Fat: 18g

- Carbohydrates: 28g

- Protein: 4g

Grilled Portobello Mushrooms with Herb Salad

Ingredients:

- 2 large Portobello mushrooms, stems removed

- 1 tablespoon olive oil

- 1 tablespoon balsamic vinegar

- Salt and pepper to taste

- 2 cups mixed salad greens

- 1/4 cup fresh herbs (parsley, cilantro, chives), chopped

- 1 tablespoon lemon juice

Directions:

1. Preheat a grill or grill pan over medium heat.

2. Brush the mushrooms with olive oil and balsamic vinegar, and season with salt and pepper.

3. Grill the mushrooms for 5-7 minutes per side, until tender and slightly charred.

4. In a large bowl, toss the salad greens with fresh herbs and lemon juice.

5. Slice the grilled mushrooms and serve them on top of the herb salad.

Nutritional Values:

- Calories: 180

- Fat: 12g

- Carbohydrates: 12g

- Protein: 4g

Cold Soba Noodle Salad with Edamame and Ginger Dressing

Ingredients:

- 4 oz soba noodles

- 1 cup shelled edamame

- 1 carrot, julienned

- 1 cucumber, julienned

- 1 tablespoon soy sauce or tamari

- 1 tablespoon rice vinegar

- 1 teaspoon grated fresh ginger

- 1 teaspoon sesame oil

- Optional: sesame seeds for topping

Directions:

1. Cook the soba noodles according to package instructions. Drain and rinse under cold water.

2. In a large bowl, combine the cooked soba noodles, edamame, carrot, and cucumber.

3. In a small bowl, whisk together the soy sauce, rice vinegar, ginger, and sesame oil.

4. Pour the dressing over the soba noodle mixture and toss to combine.

5. Serve chilled, garnished with sesame seeds if desired.

Nutritional Values:

- Calories: 300

- Fat: 8g

- Carbohydrates: 50g

- Protein: 12g

Egg Salad with Avocado and Spring Onion

Ingredients:

- 3 hard-boiled eggs, chopped

- 1/2 avocado, diced

- 1 spring onion, thinly sliced

- 1 tablespoon Greek yogurt or mayonnaise

- Salt and pepper to taste

Directions:

1. In a medium bowl, combine the chopped eggs, diced avocado, and sliced spring onion.

2. Stir in the Greek yogurt or mayonnaise until well combined.

3. Season with salt and pepper to taste.

4. Serve immediately or refrigerate for later use.

Nutritional Values:

- Calories: 250

- Fat: 20g

- Carbohydrates: 4g

- Protein: 12g

Carrot and Apple Slaw with Walnuts

Ingredients:

- 2 large carrots, grated

- 1 apple, julienned

- 1/4 cup walnuts, chopped

- 1 tablespoon lemon juice

- 1 tablespoon olive oil

- Salt and pepper to taste

Directions:

1. In a large bowl, combine the grated carrots, julienned apple, and chopped walnuts.

2. In a small bowl, whisk together the lemon juice and olive oil.

3. Pour the dressing over the carrot and apple mixture and toss to combine.

4. Season with salt and pepper to taste.

5. Serve chilled.

Nutritional Values:

- Calories: 200

- Fat: 14g

- Carbohydrates: 18g

- Protein: 3g

Baked Trout with Walnut and Parsley Crust

Ingredients:

- 2 trout fillets

- 1/4 cup walnuts, finely chopped

- 1/4 cup fresh parsley, chopped

- 1 tablespoon olive oil

- Salt and pepper to taste

- 1 lemon, sliced

Directions:

1. Preheat the oven to 375°F (190°C).

2. In a small bowl, combine the chopped walnuts, parsley, and olive oil.

3. Place the trout fillets on a baking sheet lined with parchment paper. Season with salt and pepper.

4. Press the walnut and parsley mixture onto the top of each fillet.

5. Bake for 15-20 minutes, or until the trout is cooked through and flakes easily with a fork.

6. Serve with lemon slices.

Nutritional Values:

- Calories: 300

- Fat: 20g

- Carbohydrates: 4g

- Protein: 25g

Spinach and Feta Stuffed Chicken Breast

Ingredients:

- 2 chicken breasts
- 1 cup fresh spinach, chopped
- 1/4 cup feta cheese, crumbled
- 1 tablespoon olive oil
- Salt and pepper to taste
- Optional: toothpicks to secure the chicken

Directions:

1. Preheat the oven to 375°F (190°C).
2. Slice each chicken breast horizontally to create a pocket, being careful not to cut all the way through.
3. In a small bowl, combine the chopped spinach and feta cheese.
4. Stuff each chicken breast with the spinach and feta mixture. Secure with toothpicks if necessary.
5. Heat olive oil in a skillet over medium heat. Sear the chicken breasts on both sides until golden brown, about 3-4 minutes per side.
6. Transfer the chicken breasts to a baking dish and bake for 20-25 minutes, or until the chicken is cooked through.
7. Serve hot.

Nutritional Values:

- Calories: 320
- Fat: 18g
- Carbohydrates: 2g
- Protein: 38g

Pearl Barley Risotto with Asparagus and Lemon Zest

Ingredients:

- 1 cup pearl barley
- 1 onion, diced
- 1 garlic clove, minced
- 1 tablespoon olive oil
- 4 cups vegetable broth
- 1 bunch asparagus, trimmed and cut into 1-inch pieces
- 1/4 cup grated Parmesan cheese
- Zest of 1 lemon
- Salt and pepper to taste

Directions:

1. Heat olive oil in a large skillet over medium heat. Add the onion and garlic, and cook until softened, about 5 minutes.
2. Stir in the pearl barley and cook for another 2 minutes, until lightly toasted.
3. Add the vegetable broth, 1 cup at a time, stirring frequently, until the

barley is tender and creamy, about 30 minutes.

4. Meanwhile, steam or blanch the asparagus until tender, about 3-4 minutes.

5. Stir the cooked asparagus, Parmesan cheese, and lemon zest into the risotto.

6. Season with salt and pepper to taste, and serve hot.

Nutritional Values:

- Calories: 350

- Fat: 10g

- Carbohydrates: 58g

- Protein: 12g

Gazpacho with Fresh Cucumber and Bell Pepper

Ingredients:

- 4 large tomatoes, chopped

- 1 cucumber, peeled and chopped

- 1 red bell pepper, chopped

- 1/4 cup red onion, chopped

- 2 garlic cloves, minced

- 2 tablespoons olive oil

- 1 tablespoon red wine vinegar

- Salt and pepper to taste

Directions:

1. In a blender or food processor, combine the tomatoes, cucumber, bell pepper, red onion, and garlic.

2. Blend until smooth, adding a little water if needed to reach your desired consistency.

3. Stir in the olive oil, red wine vinegar, salt, and pepper.

4. Chill the gazpacho in the refrigerator for at least 1 hour before serving.

5. Serve cold, garnished with additional chopped vegetables if desired.

Nutritional Values:

- Calories: 150

- Fat: 10g

- Carbohydrates: 15g

- Protein: 2g

CHAPTER 4

DINNER RECIPES

Grilled Turkey Burgers with Oatmeal and Herbs

Ingredients:

- 1 lb ground turkey
- 1/2 cup rolled oats
- 1 egg, beaten
- 1/4 cup fresh parsley, chopped
- 1 tablespoon fresh thyme, chopped
- 1 garlic clove, minced
- Salt and pepper to taste
- 1 tablespoon olive oil (for grilling)

Directions:

1. In a large bowl, combine the ground turkey, rolled oats, beaten egg, parsley, thyme, garlic, salt, and pepper. Mix until well combined.
2. Shape the mixture into four patties.
3. Heat a grill or grill pan over medium heat and lightly brush with olive oil.
4. Grill the turkey burgers for about 5-6 minutes per side, or until fully cooked and the internal temperature reaches 165°F (74°C).
5. Serve the burgers on whole grain buns or with a side of vegetables.

Nutritional Values:

- Calories: 250
- Fat: 12g
- Carbohydrates: 10g
- Protein: 28g

Roasted Chicken with Root Vegetables

Ingredients:

- 1 whole chicken (about 4 lbs)
- 2 carrots, peeled and chopped
- 2 parsnips, peeled and chopped
- 1 onion, quartered
- 4 garlic cloves, smashed
- 2 tablespoons olive oil

- 1 tablespoon fresh rosemary, chopped

- 1 tablespoon fresh thyme, chopped

- Salt and pepper to taste

Directions:

1. Preheat the oven to 375°F (190°C).

2. Place the chicken in a large roasting pan. Arrange the carrots, parsnips, onion, and garlic around the chicken.

3. Drizzle the olive oil over the chicken and vegetables. Sprinkle with rosemary, thyme, salt, and pepper.

4. Roast the chicken for 1 1/2 to 2 hours, or until the internal temperature reaches 165°F (74°C) and the juices run clear.

5. Let the chicken rest for 10 minutes before carving. Serve with the roasted vegetables.

Nutritional Values:

- Calories: 400

- Fat: 24g

- Carbohydrates: 15g

- Protein: 30g

Baked Haddock with a Crust of Herbs and Almonds

Ingredients:

- 4 haddock fillets

- 1/4 cup almonds, finely chopped

- 1/4 cup fresh parsley, chopped

- 1 tablespoon fresh dill, chopped

- 1 tablespoon lemon zest

- 2 tablespoons olive oil

- Salt and pepper to taste

Directions:

1. Preheat the oven to 400°F (200°C).

2. In a small bowl, combine the chopped almonds, parsley, dill, lemon zest, olive oil, salt, and pepper.

3. Place the haddock fillets on a baking sheet lined with parchment paper. Press the almond and herb mixture onto the top of each fillet.

4. Bake for 12-15 minutes, or until the fish is cooked through and flakes easily with a fork.

5. Serve with lemon wedges and a side of vegetables.

Nutritional Values:

- Calories: 320

- Fat: 20g

- Carbohydrates: 6g

- Protein: 28g

Vegan Chili with Quinoa and Black Beans

Ingredients:

- 1 cup quinoa, rinsed

- 1 can black beans, drained and rinsed

- 1 can diced tomatoes

- 1 onion, diced

- 2 garlic cloves, minced

- 1 bell pepper, diced

- 1 tablespoon chili powder

- 1 teaspoon ground cumin

- 1/4 teaspoon cayenne pepper (optional)

- 2 cups vegetable broth

- Salt and pepper to taste

- Optional: avocado slices, cilantro for garnish

Directions:

1. In a large pot, heat olive oil over medium heat. Add the onion, garlic, and bell pepper, and cook until softened, about 5 minutes.

2. Stir in the chili powder, cumin, and cayenne pepper. Cook for another minute until fragrant.

3. Add the quinoa, black beans, diced tomatoes, and vegetable broth. Bring to a boil, then reduce heat and simmer for 20-25 minutes, until the quinoa is tender.

4. Season with salt and pepper to taste. Serve hot, garnished with avocado slices and cilantro if desired.

Nutritional Values:

- Calories: 350

- Fat: 8g

- Carbohydrates: 55g

- Protein: 12g

Zucchini Noodles with Tomato Sauce and Fresh Basil

Ingredients:

- 4 medium zucchinis, spiralized into noodles

- 2 cups tomato sauce

- 1 garlic clove, minced

- 1 tablespoon olive oil

- 1/4 cup fresh basil leaves, chopped

- Salt and pepper to taste

- Optional: grated Parmesan cheese

Directions:

1. In a large skillet, heat olive oil over medium heat. Add the garlic and cook until fragrant, about 1 minute.

2. Pour in the tomato sauce and bring to a simmer. Cook for 5-7 minutes, stirring occasionally.

3. Add the zucchini noodles to the skillet and toss to combine. Cook for 2-3 minutes, until the noodles are tender but still firm.

4. Stir in the fresh basil and season with salt and pepper.

5. Serve hot, with grated Parmesan cheese if desired.

Nutritional Values:

- Calories: 180
- Fat: 8g
- Carbohydrates: 24g
- Protein: 4g

Eggplant Parmesan Lightened Up

Ingredients:

- 2 medium eggplants, sliced into 1/2-inch rounds
- 1 cup whole wheat breadcrumbs
- 1/2 cup grated Parmesan cheese
- 1 cup marinara sauce
- 1 cup shredded mozzarella cheese
- 1 tablespoon olive oil
- Salt and pepper to taste
- Optional: fresh basil for garnish

Directions:

1. Preheat the oven to 375°F (190°C). Lightly grease a baking sheet with olive oil.

2. In a shallow bowl, mix together the breadcrumbs and grated Parmesan cheese.

3. Dip each eggplant slice in the breadcrumb mixture, pressing lightly to adhere.

4. Place the breaded eggplant slices on the baking sheet and bake for 25-30 minutes, flipping halfway through, until golden brown and tender.

5. In a baking dish, layer the baked eggplant slices with marinara sauce and shredded mozzarella cheese.

6. Bake for an additional 15 minutes, or until the cheese is melted and bubbly.

7. Serve hot, garnished with fresh basil if desired.

Nutritional Values:

- Calories: 300
- Fat: 14g
- Carbohydrates: 34g
- Protein: 12g

Beef and Vegetable Stew with Thyme

Ingredients:

- 1 lb beef stew meat, cubed
- 2 carrots, sliced
- 2 potatoes, diced
- 1 onion, chopped
- 2 garlic cloves, minced
- 1 tablespoon olive oil
- 1 tablespoon fresh thyme, chopped
- 4 cups beef broth
- Salt and pepper to taste

Directions:

1. In a large pot, heat olive oil over medium heat. Add the beef cubes and brown on all sides, about 5-7 minutes.
2. Remove the beef and set aside. Add the onion and garlic to the pot and cook until softened, about 5 minutes.
3. Return the beef to the pot, along with the carrots, potatoes, thyme, and beef broth.
4. Bring to a boil, then reduce heat and simmer for 1 1/2 to 2 hours, or until the beef is tender and the vegetables are cooked through.
5. Season with salt and pepper to taste. Serve hot.

Nutritional Values:

- Calories: 350
- Fat: 14g
- Carbohydrates: 28g
- Protein: 28g

Spinach and Mushroom Lasagna

Ingredients:

- 9 whole wheat lasagna noodles
- 2 cups ricotta cheese
- 2 cups fresh spinach, chopped
- 1 cup mushrooms, sliced
- 2 cups marinara sauce
- 2 cups shredded mozzarella cheese
- 1 tablespoon olive oil
- Salt and pepper to taste

Directions:

1. Preheat the oven to 375°F (190°C).
2. Cook the lasagna noodles according to package instructions. Drain and set aside.
3. In a large skillet, heat olive oil over medium heat. Add the mushrooms and cook until tender, about 5 minutes. Stir in the spinach and

cook until wilted. Season with salt and pepper.

4. In a large baking dish, spread a layer of marinara sauce. Place three lasagna noodles on top, followed by a layer of ricotta cheese, spinach and mushroom mixture, and shredded mozzarella cheese.

5. Repeat the layers two more times, finishing with a layer of marinara sauce and mozzarella cheese.

6. Cover with foil and bake for 25 minutes. Remove the foil and bake for an additional 10 minutes, until the cheese is melted and bubbly.

7. Let the lasagna cool for 10 minutes before serving.

Nutritional Values:

- Calories: 400
- Fat: 18g
- Carbohydrates: 42g
- Protein: 22g

Cauliflower Steak with Olive Relish

Ingredients:

- 1 large head of cauliflower, cut into 1-inch thick steaks
- 1/4 cup olive oil
- 1/2 cup green olives, chopped
- 1/4 cup fresh parsley, chopped
- 1 tablespoon capers, rinsed
- 1 tablespoon lemon juice
- Salt and pepper to taste

Directions:

1. Preheat the oven to 400°F (200°C).

2. Brush the cauliflower steaks with olive oil and season with salt and pepper.

3. Place the cauliflower on a baking sheet and roast for 25-30 minutes, until tender and golden brown.

4. In a small bowl, combine the chopped olives, parsley, capers, lemon juice, and 1 tablespoon of olive oil. Stir to combine.

5. Serve the cauliflower steaks topped with the olive relish.

Nutritional Values:

- Calories: 220
- Fat: 18g
- Carbohydrates: 14g
- Protein: 4g

Seared Scallops with Sweet Corn Puree

Ingredients:

- 12 large sea scallops
- 1 tablespoon olive oil
- 2 cups fresh or frozen corn kernels

- 1/4 cup heavy cream

- 1 tablespoon butter

- Salt and pepper to taste

- Optional: fresh chives for garnish

Directions:

1. In a small saucepan, combine the corn kernels, heavy cream, and butter. Cook over medium heat for 5-7 minutes, until the corn is tender.

2. Use an immersion blender or transfer the mixture to a blender to puree until smooth. Season with salt and pepper. Keep warm.

3. Pat the scallops dry and season with salt and pepper.

4. Heat olive oil in a large skillet over medium-high heat. Sear the scallops for 2-3 minutes per side, until golden brown and cooked through.

5. Serve the scallops over the sweet corn puree, garnished with fresh chives if desired.

Nutritional Values:

- Calories: 320

- Fat: 20g

- Carbohydrates: 18g

- Protein: 18g

Stir-Fried Tofu with Broccoli and Peppers

Ingredients:

- 1 block firm tofu, drained and cubed

- 2 cups broccoli florets

- 1 red bell pepper, sliced

- 2 tablespoons soy sauce or tamari

- 1 tablespoon olive oil

- 1 garlic clove, minced

- 1 teaspoon grated ginger

- Salt and pepper to taste

Directions:

1. Heat olive oil in a large skillet over medium heat. Add the tofu cubes and cook until golden brown on all sides, about 5-7 minutes.

2. Remove the tofu from the skillet and set aside. Add the garlic and ginger to the skillet and cook until fragrant, about 1 minute.

3. Add the broccoli and bell pepper to the skillet and stir-fry for 5-7 minutes, until the vegetables are tender but still crisp.

4. Return the tofu to the skillet and add the soy sauce or tamari. Toss to combine and cook for an additional 2 minutes.

5. Serve hot.

Nutritional Values:

- Calories: 280
- Fat: 16g
- Carbohydrates: 16g
- Protein: 18g

Lentil and Vegetable Pie

Ingredients:

- 1 cup lentils, rinsed
- 2 carrots, diced
- 1 onion, chopped
- 2 garlic cloves, minced
- 1 tablespoon olive oil
- 2 cups vegetable broth
- 1 cup frozen peas
- 1/4 cup fresh parsley, chopped
- 2 potatoes, peeled and mashed
- Salt and pepper to taste

Directions:

1. Preheat the oven to 375°F (190°C).
2. In a large pot, heat olive oil over medium heat. Add the onion, carrots, and garlic, and cook until softened, about 5 minutes.
3. Stir in the lentils and vegetable broth. Bring to a boil, then reduce heat and simmer for 20-25 minutes, until the lentils are tender.
4. Stir in the peas and parsley, and season with salt and pepper.
5. Transfer the lentil mixture to a baking dish and spread the mashed potatoes on top.
6. Bake for 25-30 minutes, until the potatoes are golden brown.
7. Serve hot.

Nutritional Values:

- Calories: 320
- Fat: 8g
- Carbohydrates: 50g
- Protein: 12g

Moroccan Tagine with Chickpeas and Apricots

Ingredients:

- 1 can chickpeas, drained and rinsed
- 1 onion, diced
- 2 garlic cloves, minced
- 1 carrot, sliced
- 1 zucchini, sliced
- 1/2 cup dried apricots, chopped
- 1 tablespoon olive oil
- 1 teaspoon ground cumin
- 1/2 teaspoon ground cinnamon
- 1/4 teaspoon ground ginger
- 2 cups vegetable broth

- Salt and pepper to taste

Directions:

1. In a large pot, heat olive oil over medium heat. Add the onion and garlic, and cook until softened, about 5 minutes.

2. Stir in the cumin, cinnamon, and ginger, and cook for another minute until fragrant.

3. Add the chickpeas, carrot, zucchini, dried apricots, and vegetable broth. Bring to a boil, then reduce heat and simmer for 20-25 minutes, until the vegetables are tender.

4. Season with salt and pepper to taste. Serve hot.

Nutritional Values:

- Calories: 280
- Fat: 8g
- Carbohydrates: 48g
- Protein: 8g

Cod en Papillote with Vegetables and Pesto

Ingredients:

- 2 cod fillets
- 1 zucchini, sliced
- 1 carrot, julienned
- 1/2 red bell pepper, sliced
- 2 tablespoons pesto
- 2 tablespoons olive oil
- Salt and pepper to taste

Directions:

1. Preheat the oven to 400°F (200°C).

2. Cut two large pieces of parchment paper. Place a cod fillet in the center of each piece of paper.

3. Arrange the zucchini, carrot, and bell pepper around the cod fillets. Drizzle with olive oil and season with salt and pepper.

4. Spoon a tablespoon of pesto over each cod fillet.

5. Fold the parchment paper over the fish and vegetables to create a sealed packet.

6. Place the packets on a baking sheet and bake for 15-20 minutes, until the fish is cooked through and flakes easily with a fork.

7. Serve hot.

Nutritional Values:

- Calories: 280
- Fat: 16g
- Carbohydrates: 8g
- Protein: 24g

Stuffed Acorn Squash with Barley and Cranberries

Ingredients:

- 2 acorn squashes, halved and seeds removed

- 1 cup cooked barley

- 1/4 cup dried cranberries

- 1/4 cup chopped walnuts

- 1 tablespoon olive oil

- 1/2 teaspoon ground cinnamon

- Salt and pepper to taste

Directions:

1. Preheat the oven to 375°F (190°C).

2. Place the acorn squash halves on a baking sheet, cut side up. Drizzle with olive oil and season with salt and pepper.

3. Roast for 30-35 minutes, until the squash is tender.

4. In a large bowl, combine the cooked barley, dried cranberries, chopped walnuts, and cinnamon.

5. Spoon the barley mixture into the roasted squash halves.

6. Return to the oven and bake for an additional 10 minutes.

7. Serve hot.

Nutritional Values:

- Calories: 300

- Fat: 12g

- Carbohydrates: 46g

- Protein: 6g

Sweet and Sour Chicken with Pineapple

Ingredients:

- 1 lb chicken breast, cut into bite-sized pieces

- 1/2 cup pineapple chunks

- 1 bell pepper, sliced

- 1 onion, sliced

- 1/4 cup apple cider vinegar

- 2 tablespoons honey

- 1 tablespoon soy sauce or tamari

- 1 tablespoon olive oil

- 1 teaspoon cornstarch (optional, for thickening)

- Salt and pepper to taste

Directions:

1. In a large skillet, heat olive oil over medium heat. Add the chicken pieces and cook until browned on all sides, about 5-7 minutes.

2. Add the onion and bell pepper to the skillet and cook until softened, about 5 minutes.

3. Stir in the pineapple chunks, apple cider vinegar, honey, and soy sauce or tamari.

4. If desired, mix the cornstarch with a little water and stir it into the sauce to thicken.

5. Cook for another 3-4 minutes, until the sauce is thickened and the chicken is cooked through.

6. Serve hot.

Nutritional Values:

- Calories: 320
- Fat: 10g
- Carbohydrates: 30g
- Protein: 28g

Miso Soup with Tofu and Seaweed

Ingredients:

- 4 cups water
- 2 tablespoons miso paste
- 1/2 block firm tofu, cubed
- 1/4 cup dried seaweed (wakame)
- 1 green onion, sliced
- 1 tablespoon soy sauce or tamari

Directions:

1. In a medium pot, bring water to a simmer. Stir in the miso paste until dissolved.

2. Add the cubed tofu and dried seaweed to the pot. Simmer for 5-7 minutes, until the seaweed is rehydrated and the tofu is heated through.

3. Stir in the soy sauce or tamari and sliced green onion.

4. Serve hot.

Nutritional Values:

- Calories: 120
- Fat: 6g
- Carbohydrates: 8g
- Protein: 10g

Pasta Primavera with Whole Wheat Pasta

Ingredients:

- 8 oz whole wheat pasta
- 1 zucchini, sliced
- 1 bell pepper, sliced
- 1 carrot, julienned
- 1 cup cherry tomatoes, halved
- 2 garlic cloves, minced
- 2 tablespoons olive oil
- 1/4 cup grated Parmesan cheese
- Salt and pepper to taste
- Optional: fresh basil for garnish

Directions:

1. Cook the pasta according to package instructions. Drain and set aside.

2. In a large skillet, heat olive oil over medium heat. Add the garlic and cook until fragrant, about 1 minute.

3. Add the zucchini, bell pepper, and carrot to the skillet. Stir-fry for 5-7 minutes, until the vegetables are tender but still crisp.

4. Stir in the cherry tomatoes and cooked pasta. Toss to combine and cook for another 2 minutes.

5. Remove from heat and stir in the grated Parmesan cheese.

6. Season with salt and pepper, and garnish with fresh basil if desired.

7. Serve hot.

Nutritional Values:

- Calories: 320
- Fat: 12g
- Carbohydrates: 48g
- Protein: 10g

Shepherd's Pie with Lentils and Sweet Potato

Ingredients:

- 1 cup lentils, rinsed
- 2 carrots, diced
- 1 onion, chopped
- 2 garlic cloves, minced
- 1 tablespoon olive oil
- 2 cups vegetable broth
- 1 cup frozen peas
- 4 sweet potatoes, peeled and mashed
- 1 tablespoon butter
- Salt and pepper to taste

Directions:

1. Preheat the oven to 375°F (190°C).

2. In a large pot, heat olive oil over medium heat. Add the onion, carrots, and garlic, and cook until softened, about 5 minutes.

3. Stir in the lentils and vegetable broth. Bring to a boil, then reduce heat and simmer for 20-25 minutes, until the lentils are tender.

4. Stir in the peas and season with salt and pepper.

5. Transfer the lentil mixture to a baking dish and spread the mashed sweet potatoes on top.

6. Dot the sweet potatoes with butter.

7. Bake for 25-30 minutes, until the top is golden brown.

8. Serve hot.

Nutritional Values:

- Calories: 350
- Fat: 10g
- Carbohydrates: 58g
- Protein: 12g

Ratatouille with Eggplant, Zucchini, and Tomato

Ingredients:

- 1 eggplant, diced

- 1 zucchini, sliced

- 1 bell pepper, diced

- 4 tomatoes, chopped

- 1 onion, diced

- 2 garlic cloves, minced

- 2 tablespoons olive oil

- 1 teaspoon dried thyme

- Salt and pepper to taste

Directions:

1. In a large pot, heat olive oil over medium heat. Add the onion and garlic, and cook until softened, about 5 minutes.

2. Stir in the eggplant, zucchini, and bell pepper. Cook for another 5-7 minutes, until the vegetables begin to soften.

3. Add the chopped tomatoes, dried thyme, salt, and pepper. Bring to a simmer and cook for 15-20 minutes, until the vegetables are tender and the flavors are well combined.

4. Serve hot or at room temperature.

Nutritional Values:

- Calories: 220

- Fat: 14g

- Carbohydrates: 24g

- Protein: 4g

Grilled Shrimp with Mango Salsa

Ingredients:

- 1 lb shrimp, peeled and deveined

- 1 tablespoon olive oil

- 1 mango, diced

- 1/4 red onion, diced

- 1/4 cup fresh cilantro, chopped

- 1 tablespoon lime juice

- Salt and pepper to taste

Directions:

1. Preheat a grill or grill pan over medium heat.

2. Toss the shrimp with olive oil, salt, and pepper.

3. Grill the shrimp for 2-3 minutes per side, until pink and opaque.

4. In a medium bowl, combine the diced mango, red onion, cilantro, and lime juice. Stir to combine.

5. Serve the grilled shrimp topped with mango salsa.

Nutritional Values:

- Calories: 240

- Fat: 8g

- Carbohydrates: 16g

- Protein: 28g

Frittata with Kale, Potatoes, and Feta

Ingredients:

- 6 large eggs
- 1 cup kale, chopped
- 1 potato, diced
- 1/4 cup feta cheese, crumbled
- 1 tablespoon olive oil
- Salt and pepper to taste

Directions:

1. Preheat the oven to 375°F (190°C).
2. In a large, oven-safe skillet, heat olive oil over medium heat. Add the diced potato and cook until tender, about 10 minutes.
3. Stir in the chopped kale and cook until wilted, about 3 minutes.
4. In a bowl, whisk the eggs and season with salt and pepper.
5. Pour the eggs over the vegetables in the skillet. Sprinkle the feta cheese on top.
6. Transfer the skillet to the oven and bake for 10-12 minutes, until the eggs are set.
7. Serve hot.

Nutritional Values:

- Calories: 250
- Fat: 16g
- Carbohydrates: 12g
- Protein: 16g

Vegetarian Paella with Bell Peppers and Lima Beans

Ingredients:

- 1 cup arborio rice
- 1 onion, diced
- 1 bell pepper, sliced
- 1 cup lima beans, cooked
- 2 garlic cloves, minced
- 1 tablespoon olive oil
- 1/4 teaspoon saffron threads
- 4 cups vegetable broth
- Salt and pepper to taste

Directions:

1. Heat olive oil in a large skillet over medium heat. Add the onion, bell pepper, and garlic, and cook until softened, about 5 minutes.
2. Stir in the arborio rice and saffron, and cook for another 2 minutes, until the rice is lightly toasted.
3. Add the vegetable broth and bring to a boil. Reduce heat to low, cover, and simmer for 15 minutes.
4. Stir in the cooked lima beans and continue to cook for another 10

minutes, until the rice is tender and the liquid is absorbed.

5. Season with salt and pepper to taste, and serve hot.

Nutritional Values:

- Calories: 300

- Fat: 8g

- Carbohydrates: 55g

- Protein: 7g

Roasted Pork Tenderloin with Apples and Onions

Ingredients:

- 1 pork tenderloin (about 1 lb)

- 2 apples, sliced

- 1 onion, sliced

- 2 tablespoons olive oil

- 1 tablespoon fresh rosemary, chopped

- Salt and pepper to taste

Directions:

1. Preheat the oven to 375°F (190°C).

2. In a large oven-safe skillet, heat olive oil over medium heat. Season the pork tenderloin with salt, pepper, and rosemary.

3. Sear the pork on all sides until browned, about 5-7 minutes.

4. Add the sliced apples and onions to the skillet around the pork.

5. Transfer the skillet to the oven and roast for 20-25 minutes, or until the pork reaches an internal temperature of 145°F (63°C).

6. Let the pork rest for 5 minutes before slicing. Serve with the roasted apples and onions.

Nutritional Values:

- Calories: 350

- Fat: 16g

- Carbohydrates: 20g

- Protein: 32g

Wild Rice and Turkey Casserole

Ingredients:

- 1 cup wild rice, cooked

- 2 cups cooked turkey, shredded

- 1 onion, diced

- 1 celery stalk, diced

- 1 carrot, diced

- 1/2 cup mushrooms, sliced

- 1 cup chicken broth

- 1/2 cup shredded cheddar cheese

- 1 tablespoon olive oil

- Salt and pepper to taste

Directions:

1. Preheat the oven to 350°F (175°C).

2. In a large skillet, heat olive oil over medium heat. Add the onion, celery, carrot, and mushrooms, and cook until softened, about 5 minutes.

3. Stir in the cooked wild rice and shredded turkey. Season with salt and pepper.

4. Pour in the chicken broth and stir to combine.

5. Transfer the mixture to a baking dish and sprinkle the shredded cheddar cheese on top.

6. Bake for 20-25 minutes, until the cheese is melted and bubbly.

7. Serve hot.

Nutritional Values:

- Calories: 380
- Fat: 16g
- Carbohydrates: 32g
- Protein: 28g

As you reach the midpoint of "Diverticulitis Diet After 60," we would love to hear your thoughts on the journey so far. Your insights are invaluable to us and help other readers understand the benefits of following the advice laid out in these pages.

How You Can Share Your Review:

Through Amazon.com:

- Go to the Amazon page where you found my book.

- Navigate to the 'Customer Reviews' section.

- Click on 'Write a customer review' to share your valuable insights.

Instant QR Code Access: Simply scan the QR code below with your smartphone to be directed to the Amazon review section.

CHAPTER 5

SNACKS RECIPES

Hummus with Carrot and Celery Sticks

Ingredients:

- 1 can chickpeas, drained and rinsed
- 2 tablespoons tahini
- 2 tablespoons olive oil
- 1 garlic clove, minced
- Juice of 1 lemon
- Salt and pepper to taste
- 2 carrots, cut into sticks
- 2 celery stalks, cut into sticks

Directions:

1. In a food processor, combine the chickpeas, tahini, olive oil, garlic, lemon juice, salt, and pepper. Blend until smooth, adding a little water if needed to reach your desired consistency.
2. Transfer the hummus to a serving bowl.
3. Serve with carrot and celery sticks.

Nutritional Values:

- Calories: 220
- Fat: 14g
- Carbohydrates: 20g
- Protein: 6g

Greek Yogurt with Honey and Walnut

Ingredients:

- 1 cup plain Greek yogurt
- 1 tablespoon honey
- 1/4 cup walnuts, chopped

Directions:

1. Spoon the Greek yogurt into a serving bowl.
2. Drizzle the honey over the yogurt.
3. Sprinkle the chopped walnuts on top.
4. Serve immediately.

Nutritional Values:

- Calories: 250
- Fat: 12g

- Carbohydrates: 20g
- Protein: 15g

Baked Kale Chips

Ingredients:

- 1 bunch kale, stems removed and leaves torn into bite-sized pieces
- 1 tablespoon olive oil
- 1/4 teaspoon salt

Directions:

1. Preheat the oven to 300°F (150°C).
2. In a large bowl, toss the kale pieces with olive oil and salt until evenly coated.
3. Spread the kale on a baking sheet in a single layer.
4. Bake for 20-25 minutes, or until the kale is crispy and slightly browned.
5. Serve immediately.

Nutritional Values:

- Calories: 80
- Fat: 7g
- Carbohydrates: 4g
- Protein: 2g

Almond and Date Energy Balls

Ingredients:

- 1 cup almonds
- 1 cup pitted dates
- 1 tablespoon cocoa powder
- 1 teaspoon vanilla extract
- 1 tablespoon water (if needed)

Directions:

1. In a food processor, combine the almonds, dates, cocoa powder, and vanilla extract. Blend until the mixture is well combined and sticks together. Add a little water if needed.
2. Roll the mixture into small balls.
3. Store in an airtight container in the refrigerator.

Nutritional Values:

- Calories: 100 per ball
- Fat: 5g
- Carbohydrates: 12g
- Protein: 2g

Cottage Cheese with Sliced Tomato and Cracked Pepper

Ingredients:

- 1/2 cup cottage cheese
- 1 small tomato, sliced
- Cracked black pepper to taste

Directions:

1. Spoon the cottage cheese into a serving bowl.

2. Top with sliced tomato.

3. Sprinkle with cracked black pepper.

4. Serve immediately.

Nutritional Values:

- Calories: 120

- Fat: 3g

- Carbohydrates: 6g

- Protein: 14g

Apple Slices with Almond Butter

Ingredients:

- 1 apple, sliced

- 2 tablespoons almond butter

Directions:

1. Arrange the apple slices on a plate.

2. Serve with almond butter for dipping.

3. Serve immediately.

Nutritional Values:

- Calories: 200

- Fat: 10g

- Carbohydrates: 28g

- Protein: 4g

Spiced Roasted Chickpeas

Ingredients:

- 1 can chickpeas, drained and rinsed

- 1 tablespoon olive oil

- 1/2 teaspoon ground cumin

- 1/2 teaspoon smoked paprika

- 1/4 teaspoon salt

Directions:

1. Preheat the oven to 400°F (200°C).

2. In a large bowl, toss the chickpeas with olive oil, cumin, smoked paprika, and salt.

3. Spread the chickpeas on a baking sheet in a single layer.

4. Roast for 20-25 minutes, stirring halfway through, until crispy.

5. Serve immediately.

Nutritional Values:

- Calories: 160

- Fat: 7g

- Carbohydrates: 18g

- Protein: 6g

Guacamole with Whole Grain Crackers

Ingredients:

- 2 ripe avocados, peeled and mashed

- 1/4 cup red onion, diced
- 1 small tomato, diced
- Juice of 1 lime
- Salt and pepper to taste
- Whole grain crackers for serving

Directions:

1. In a bowl, combine the mashed avocados, red onion, tomato, lime juice, salt, and pepper. Mix well.

2. Serve the guacamole with whole grain crackers.

Nutritional Values:

- Calories: 200 per serving (guacamole only)
- Fat: 18g
- Carbohydrates: 10g
- Protein: 2g

Stuffed Cherry Tomatoes with Herbed Goat Cheese

Ingredients:

- 12 cherry tomatoes
- 1/4 cup goat cheese
- 1 tablespoon fresh herbs (such as basil, parsley, or chives), chopped

Directions:

1. Slice the tops off the cherry tomatoes and scoop out the seeds.

2. In a small bowl, mix the goat cheese with the chopped herbs.

3. Fill each tomato with the herbed goat cheese.

4. Serve immediately.

Nutritional Values:

- Calories: 100 per 3 stuffed tomatoes
- Fat: 8g
- Carbohydrates: 4g
- Protein: 4g

Banana and Oat Cookies

Ingredients:

- 2 ripe bananas, mashed
- 1 cup rolled oats
- 1/4 cup raisins or chocolate chips (optional)
- 1/2 teaspoon vanilla extract

Directions:

1. Preheat the oven to 350°F (175°C).

2. In a large bowl, mix the mashed bananas, rolled oats, raisins or chocolate chips (if using), and vanilla extract until well combined.

3. Drop spoon fuls of the mixture onto a baking sheet lined with parchment paper.

4. Bake for 12-15 minutes, or until the cookies are set and lightly browned.

5. Let cool before serving.

Nutritional Values:

- Calories: 90 per cookie
- Fat: 1g
- Carbohydrates: 19g
- Protein: 2g

Mixed Nuts and Dried Fruit Trail Mix

Ingredients:

- 1/2 cup almonds
- 1/2 cup walnuts
- 1/2 cup cashews
- 1/2 cup dried cranberries
- 1/2 cup dried apricots, chopped

Directions:

1. In a large bowl, combine the almonds, walnuts, cashews, dried cranberries, and chopped dried apricots.
2. Mix well and store in an airtight container.

Nutritional Values:

- Calories: 180 per 1/4 cup serving
- Fat: 12g
- Carbohydrates: 18g
- Protein: 4g

Edamame with Sea Salt

Ingredients:

- 1 cup shelled edamame
- 1/4 teaspoon sea salt

Directions:

1. Bring a pot of water to a boil and cook the edamame for 3-5 minutes, until tender.
2. Drain the edamame and sprinkle with sea salt.
3. Serve immediately.

Nutritional Values:

- Calories: 120
- Fat: 5g
- Carbohydrates: 9g
- Protein: 11g

Cucumber Rounds with Smoked Salmon and Dill

Ingredients:

- 1 cucumber, sliced into rounds
- 4 oz smoked salmon, cut into small pieces
- Fresh dill for garnish

Directions:

1. Arrange the cucumber rounds on a serving platter.

2. Top each cucumber round with a piece of smoked salmon.

3. Garnish with fresh dill.

4. Serve immediately.

Nutritional Values:

- Calories: 150 per serving

- Fat: 8g

- Carbohydrates: 4g

- Protein: 16g

Peach and Ricotta Toast

Ingredients:

- 2 slices whole grain bread, toasted

- 1/2 cup ricotta cheese

- 1 peach, sliced

- 1 tablespoon honey

Directions:

1. Spread the ricotta cheese evenly over the toasted bread slices.

2. Top with peach slices.

3. Drizzle with honey.

4. Serve immediately.

Nutritional Values:

- Calories: 250

- Fat: 8g

- Carbohydrates: 35g

- Protein: 10g

Roasted Pumpkin Seeds with Paprika

Ingredients:

- 1 cup pumpkin seeds

- 1 tablespoon olive oil

- 1/2 teaspoon smoked paprika

- 1/4 teaspoon salt

Directions:

1. Preheat the oven to 300°F (150°C).

2. In a bowl, toss the pumpkin seeds with olive oil, smoked paprika, and salt until evenly coated.

3. Spread the seeds on a baking sheet in a single layer.

4. Bake for 20-25 minutes, stirring occasionally, until the seeds are crispy and golden brown.

5. Let cool before serving.

Nutritional Values:

- Calories: 180 per 1/4 cup serving

- Fat: 14g

- Carbohydrates: 6g

- Protein: 8g

CHAPTER 6

DESSERTS RECIPES

Baked Apples with Cinnamon and Nuts

Ingredients:

- 4 large apples, cored
- 1/4 cup chopped walnuts
- 1/4 cup raisins
- 1 tablespoon honey
- 1 teaspoon ground cinnamon
- 1 tablespoon butter

Directions:

1. Preheat the oven to 350°F (175°C).
2. In a small bowl, mix together the chopped walnuts, raisins, honey, and ground cinnamon.
3. Stuff each apple with the walnut mixture and place a small piece of butter on top.
4. Arrange the apples in a baking dish and cover with foil.
5. Bake for 25-30 minutes, until the apples are tender.
6. Serve warm.

Nutritional Values:

- Calories: 220 per apple
- Fat: 10g
- Carbohydrates: 34g
- Protein: 2g

Poached Pears in White Wine

Ingredients:

- 4 ripe pears, peeled and cored
- 2 cups white wine
- 1/2 cup sugar
- 1 cinnamon stick
- 2 cloves
- Zest of 1 lemon

Directions:

1. In a large saucepan, combine the white wine, sugar, cinnamon stick, cloves, and lemon zest. Bring to a simmer over medium heat.

2. Add the pears to the saucepan, making sure they are fully submerged in the liquid.

3. Simmer for 20-25 minutes, or until the pears are tender.

4. Remove the pears from the saucepan and set aside.

5. Continue simmering the liquid until it is reduced by half and slightly thickened.

6. Serve the pears drizzled with the reduced syrup.

Nutritional Values:

- Calories: 180 per pear

- Fat: 0g

- Carbohydrates: 30g

- Protein: 0g

Blueberry and Almond Clafoutis

Ingredients:

- 1 cup fresh blueberries

- 1/4 cup sliced almonds

- 3 large eggs

- 1/2 cup almond flour

- 1/2 cup milk (dairy or non-dairy)

- 1/4 cup honey or maple syrup

- 1 teaspoon vanilla extract

- Pinch of salt

Directions:

1. Preheat the oven to 350°F (175°C).

2. Grease a baking dish and scatter the blueberries and sliced almonds evenly across the bottom.

3. In a mixing bowl, whisk together the eggs, almond flour, milk, honey, vanilla extract, and salt until smooth.

4. Pour the batter over the blueberries and almonds.

5. Bake for 25-30 minutes, or until the clafoutis is set and golden brown.

6. Serve warm or at room temperature.

Nutritional Values:

- Calories: 220 per serving

- Fat: 12g

- Carbohydrates: 22g

- Protein: 6g

Carrot and Walnut Cake with Yogurt Frosting

Ingredients:

- 1 1/2 cups grated carrots

- 1 cup whole wheat flour

- 1/2 cup walnuts, chopped

- 1/2 cup honey or maple syrup

- 1/4 cup olive oil

- 2 large eggs

- 1 teaspoon baking powder

- 1/2 teaspoon ground cinnamon

- 1/2 teaspoon ground ginger

- Pinch of salt

- 1/2 cup Greek yogurt (for frosting)

- 1 tablespoon honey (for frosting)

Directions:

1. Preheat the oven to 350°F (175°C). Grease a cake pan.

2. In a large bowl, mix together the grated carrots, whole wheat flour, chopped walnuts, honey, olive oil, eggs, baking powder, cinnamon, ginger, and salt until well combined.

3. Pour the batter into the prepared cake pan and smooth the top.

4. Bake for 25-30 minutes, or until a toothpick inserted into the center comes out clean.

5. Allow the cake to cool completely before frosting.

6. For the frosting, mix together the Greek yogurt and honey. Spread over the cooled cake.

7. Serve immediately.

Nutritional Values:

- Calories: 280 per slice

- Fat: 14g

- Carbohydrates: 32g

- Protein: 6g

Strawberry and Chia Seed Pudding

Ingredients:

- 2 cups fresh strawberries, hulled and chopped

- 1/2 cup chia seeds

- 2 cups almond milk or other milk of choice

- 2 tablespoons honey or maple syrup

- 1 teaspoon vanilla extract

Directions:

1. In a blender, puree the strawberries until smooth.

2. In a mixing bowl, whisk together the strawberry puree, chia seeds, almond milk, honey, and vanilla extract.

3. Pour the mixture into individual serving dishes or a large bowl.

4. Refrigerate for at least 4 hours or overnight, until the chia seeds have absorbed the liquid and the pudding has thickened.

5. Serve chilled.

Nutritional Values:

- Calories: 180 per serving

- Fat: 9g

- Carbohydrates: 24g

- Protein: 5g

Coconut Rice Pudding

Ingredients:

- 1 cup jasmine rice
- 2 cups coconut milk
- 1/2 cup water
- 1/4 cup sugar
- 1 teaspoon vanilla extract
- 1/4 teaspoon ground cinnamon
- Optional: shredded coconut for topping

Directions:

1. In a large saucepan, combine the jasmine rice, coconut milk, water, sugar, vanilla extract, and cinnamon.
2. Bring to a simmer over medium heat, stirring frequently.
3. Reduce the heat to low and cook for 20-25 minutes, stirring occasionally, until the rice is tender and the mixture is creamy.
4. Serve warm, topped with shredded coconut if desired.

Nutritional Values:

- Calories: 220 per serving
- Fat: 10g
- Carbohydrates: 30g

- Protein: 3g

Dark Chocolate and Avocado Mousse

Ingredients:

- 2 ripe avocados, peeled and pitted
- 1/4 cup unsweetened cocoa powder
- 1/4 cup honey or maple syrup
- 1/4 cup almond milk or other milk of choice
- 1 teaspoon vanilla extract
- Pinch of salt

Directions:

1. In a blender or food processor, combine the avocados, cocoa powder, honey, almond milk, vanilla extract, and salt. Blend until smooth and creamy.
2. Spoon the mousse into individual serving dishes.
3. Refrigerate for at least 1 hour before serving.
4. Serve chilled.

Nutritional Values:

- Calories: 200 per serving
- Fat: 14g
- Carbohydrates: 22g
- Protein: 2g

Peach and Raspberry Crisp

Ingredients:

- 4 large peaches, sliced
- 1 cup fresh raspberries
- 1/2 cup rolled oats
- 1/4 cup almond flour
- 1/4 cup chopped almonds
- 2 tablespoons honey or maple syrup
- 2 tablespoons coconut oil, melted
- 1 teaspoon ground cinnamon

Directions:

1. Preheat the oven to 350°F (175°C).
2. In a baking dish, combine the sliced peaches and raspberries.
3. In a separate bowl, mix together the rolled oats, almond flour, chopped almonds, honey, coconut oil, and cinnamon.
4. Sprinkle the oat mixture evenly over the fruit.
5. Bake for 25-30 minutes, until the topping is golden brown and the fruit is bubbly.
6. Serve warm.

Nutritional Values:

- Calories: 250 per serving
- Fat: 12g
- Carbohydrates: 34g

Lemon and Poppy Seed Loaf

Ingredients:

- 1 1/2 cups whole wheat flour
- 1/2 cup almond flour
- 1/2 cup sugar
- 1/4 cup poppy seeds
- 1/2 teaspoon baking powder
- 1/4 teaspoon baking soda
- 1/4 teaspoon salt
- Zest of 1 lemon
- 1/2 cup almond milk or other milk of choice
- 1/4 cup lemon juice
- 1/4 cup olive oil
- 2 large eggs

Directions:

1. Preheat the oven to 350°F (175°C). Grease a loaf pan.
2. In a large bowl, whisk together the whole wheat flour, almond flour, sugar, poppy seeds, baking powder, baking soda, salt, and lemon zest.
3. In a separate bowl, whisk together the almond milk, lemon juice, olive oil, and eggs.

4. Pour the wet ingredients into the dry ingredients and mix until just combined.

5. Pour the batter into the prepared loaf pan and smooth the top.

6. Bake for 40-45 minutes, or until a toothpick inserted into the center comes out clean.

7. Allow the loaf to cool in the pan for 10 minutes before transferring to a wire rack to cool completely.

8. Serve sliced.

Nutritional Values:

- Calories: 220 per slice
- Fat: 12g
- Carbohydrates: 24g
- Protein: 5g

Grilled Pineapple with Honey and Mint

Ingredients:

- 1 fresh pineapple, peeled, cored, and sliced
- 2 tablespoons honey
- 1 tablespoon fresh mint, chopped

Directions:

1. Preheat a grill or grill pan over medium heat.

2. Grill the pineapple slices for 2-3 minutes per side, until grill marks appear and the pineapple is slightly caramelized.

3. Remove from the grill and drizzle with honey.

4. Sprinkle with chopped mint.

5. Serve warm.

Nutritional Values:

- Calories: 120 per serving
- Fat: 0g
- Carbohydrates: 31g
- Protein: 1g

Watermelon and Mint Sorbet

Ingredients:

- 4 cups watermelon, cubed and seeds removed
- 1/4 cup honey or maple syrup
- 2 tablespoons fresh mint, chopped
- Juice of 1 lime

Directions:

1. In a blender, combine the watermelon, honey, mint, and lime juice. Blend until smooth.

2. Pour the mixture into a shallow dish and freeze for 2-3 hours, stirring every 30 minutes to break up any ice crystals.

3. Once fully frozen, scoop into serving bowls.

4. Serve immediately.

Nutritional Values:

- Calories: 100 per serving

- Fat: 0g

- Carbohydrates: 25g

- Protein: 1g

Baked Figs with Honey and Cream Cheese

Ingredients:

- 8 fresh figs, halved

- 4 ounces cream cheese, softened

- 2 tablespoons honey

- 1/4 teaspoon ground cinnamon

Directions:

1. Preheat the oven to 350°F (175°C).

2. Arrange the fig halves on a baking sheet.

3. In a small bowl, mix the cream cheese with 1 tablespoon of honey and the ground cinnamon.

4. Spoon the cream cheese mixture onto the fig halves.

5. Drizzle with the remaining honey.

6. Bake for 10-12 minutes, until the figs are softened and the cheese is slightly melted.

7. Serve warm.

Nutritional Values:

- Calories: 150 per 2 fig halves

- Fat: 6g

- Carbohydrates: 24g

- Protein: 2g

Apricot and Pistachio Tart

Ingredients:

- 1 cup almond flour

- 1/4 cup coconut oil, melted

- 2 tablespoons honey

- 1/2 teaspoon vanilla extract

- 8 fresh apricots, halved and pitted

- 1/4 cup chopped pistachios

Directions:

1. Preheat the oven to 350°F (175°C).

2. In a medium bowl, mix together the almond flour, melted coconut oil, honey, and vanilla extract until a dough forms.

3. Press the dough into the bottom of a tart pan.

4. Arrange the apricot halves, cut side up, on top of the dough.

5. Sprinkle with chopped pistachios.

6. Bake for 25-30 minutes, until the tart is golden brown and the apricots are tender.

7. Let cool before serving.

Nutritional Values:

- Calories: 180 per slice
- Fat: 12g
- Carbohydrates: 16g
- Protein: 3g

Chocolate Chip and Banana Muffins

Ingredients:

- 2 ripe bananas, mashed
- 1/4 cup honey or maple syrup
- 1/4 cup olive oil
- 2 large eggs
- 1 teaspoon vanilla extract
- 1 1/2 cups whole wheat flour
- 1 teaspoon baking powder
- 1/2 teaspoon baking soda
- 1/4 teaspoon salt
- 1/2 cup dark chocolate chips

Directions:

1. Preheat the oven to 350°F (175°C). Line a muffin tin with paper liners.
2. In a large bowl, mix together the mashed bananas, honey, olive oil, eggs, and vanilla extract.
3. In a separate bowl, whisk together the whole wheat flour, baking powder, baking soda, and salt.
4. Add the dry ingredients to the wet ingredients and mix until just combined.
5. Fold in the dark chocolate chips.
6. Divide the batter evenly among the muffin cups.
7. Bake for 18-20 minutes, or until a toothpick inserted into the center comes out clean.
8. Allow the muffins to cool in the tin for 5 minutes before transferring to a wire rack to cool completely.

Nutritional Values:

- Calories: 200 per muffin
- Fat: 10g
- Carbohydrates: 26g
- Protein: 4g

Vanilla Panna Cotta with Berry Compote

Ingredients:

- 2 cups heavy cream or coconut milk
- 1/4 cup sugar
- 1 teaspoon vanilla extract
- 2 teaspoons unflavored gelatin
- 2 tablespoons cold water

- 1 cup mixed berries (strawberries, blueberries, raspberries)

- 1 tablespoon honey or maple syrup

Directions:

1. In a small bowl, sprinkle the gelatin over the cold water and let it sit for 5 minutes to bloom.

2. In a saucepan, heat the heavy cream (or coconut milk) and sugar over medium heat until the sugar is dissolved and the mixture is just about to simmer. Remove from heat.

3. Stir in the vanilla extract and the bloomed gelatin until fully dissolved.

4. Pour the mixture into individual serving dishes and refrigerate for at least 4 hours, or until set.

5. Meanwhile, prepare the berry compote by combining the mixed berries and honey in a saucepan. Cook over medium heat until the berries are softened and the mixture is slightly thickened.

6. Once the panna cotta is set, top with the berry compote.

7. Serve chilled.

Nutritional Values:

- Calories: 250 per serving

- Fat: 20g

- Carbohydrates: 18g

- Protein: 4g

CHAPTER 7

BONUS

31-Day Meal Plan (tables)

Days 1 to 10

Day	Breakfast	Lunch	Dinner	Snack	Dessert
Day 1	Oatmeal with Sliced Pears and Almond Butter	Lentil Soup with Carrots and Celery	Grilled Turkey Burgers with Oatmeal and Herbs	Greek Yogurt with Honey and Walnut	Baked Apples with Cinnamon and Nuts
Day 2	Buckwheat Pancakes with Blueberry Compote	Quinoa Tabbouleh with Cucumbers and Mint	Roasted Chicken with Root Vegetables	Baked Kale Chips	Poached Pears in White Wine
Day 3	Scrambled Eggs with Spinach and Mushrooms	Baked Salmon with Dill and Lemon	Baked Haddock with a Crust of Herbs and Almonds	Almond and Date Energy Balls	Blueberry and Almond Clafoutis
Day 4	Quinoa Porridge with	Grilled Chicken Salad with	Vegan Chili with Quinoa	Cottage Cheese with Sliced	Carrot and Walnut Cake

Day	Breakfast	Lunch	Dinner	Snack	Dessert
	Apple and Cinnamon	Mixed Greens and Avocado	and Black Beans	Tomato and Cracked Pepper	with Yogurt Frosting
Day 5	Smoothie Bowl with Banana, Kiwi, and Flaxseed	Vegetable Stir-Fry with Tofu and Tamari Sauce	Zucchini Noodles with Tomato Sauce and Fresh Basil	Apple Slices with Almond Butter	Strawberry and Chia Seed Pudding
Day 6	Chia Pudding with Coconut Milk and Mango	Turkey and Spinach Wrap with Whole Wheat Tortilla	Eggplant Parmesan Lightened Up	Spiced Roasted Chickpeas	Coconut Rice Pudding
Day 7	Barley Breakfast Salad with Citrus and Walnuts	Beetroot and Goat Cheese Arugula Salad	Beef and Vegetable Stew with Thyme	Guacamole with Whole Grain Crackers	Dark Chocolate and Avocado Mousse
Day 8	Whole Wheat Toast with Avocado and Poached Egg	Stuffed Bell Peppers with Brown Rice and Herbs	Spinach and Mushroom Lasagna	Stuffed Cherry Tomatoes with Herbed Goat Cheese	Peach and Raspberry Crisp
Day 9	Baked Sweet Potato and Kale Hash	Butternut Squash Soup with a Hint of Ginger	Cauliflower Steak with Olive Relish	Banana and Oat Cookies	Lemon and Poppy Seed Loaf

Day	Breakfast	Lunch	Dinner	Snack	Dessert
Day 10	Millet Cereal with Raisins and Honey	Pan-Seared Cod with Fennel and Orange Salad	Lentil and Vegetable Pie	Mixed Nuts and Dried Fruit Trail Mix	Grilled Pineapple with Honey and Mint

Days 11 to 20

Day	Breakfast	Lunch	Dinner	Snack	Dessert
Day 11	Rice Cakes Topped with Ricotta and Fresh Berries	Mediterranean Chickpea and Eggplant Stew	Moroccan Tagine with Chickpeas and Apricots	Edamame with Sea Salt	Watermelon and Mint Sorbet
Day 12	Sautéed Tofu with Asparagus and Tomatoes	Cauliflower Rice with Grilled Zucchini and Pesto	Cod en Papillote with Vegetables and Pesto	Cucumber Rounds with Smoked Salmon and Dill	Baked Figs with Honey and Cream Cheese
Day 13	Multigrain Waffles with Strawberry Sauce	Vegetable Paella with Saffron and Artichokes	Stuffed Acorn Squash with Barley and Cranberries	Peach and Ricotta Toast	Apricot and Pistachio Tart
Day 14	Savory Oatmeal with Grated Zucchini and Thyme	Broccoli and Purple Cabbage Coleslaw	Sweet and Sour Chicken with Pineapple	Roasted Pumpkin Seeds with Paprika	Chocolate Chip and Banana Muffins

Day	Breakfast	Lunch	Dinner	Snack	Dessert
Day 15	Cottage Cheese with Sliced Peaches and Pumpkin Seeds	Sweet Potato and Black Bean Burrito	Miso Soup with Tofu and Seaweed	Greek Yogurt with Homemade Granola and Apple Slices	Vanilla Panna Cotta with Berry Compote
Day 16	Greek Yogurt with Homemade Granola and Apple Slices	Tomato and Basil Bruschetta on Whole Grain Bread	Pasta Primavera with Whole Wheat Pasta	Baked Kale Chips	Baked Apples with Cinnamon and Nuts
Day 17	Soft-Boiled Egg with Asparagus Soldiers	Spicy Pumpkin Soup with Coconut Milk	Shepherd's Pie with Lentils and Sweet Potato	Mixed Nuts and Dried Fruit Trail Mix	Poached Pears in White Wine
Day 18	Breakfast Lentils with Carrots and Celery	Grilled Portobello Mushrooms with Herb Salad	Ratatouille with Eggplant, Zucchini, and Tomato	Almond and Date Energy Balls	Blueberry and Almond Clafoutis
Day 19	Spelt Muffins with Pear and Ginger	Cold Soba Noodle Salad with Edamame and Ginger Dressing	Grilled Shrimp with Mango Salsa	Apple Slices with Almond Butter	Carrot and Walnut Cake with Yogurt Frosting
Day 20	Polenta with Roasted	Egg Salad with Avocado and Spring Onion	Frittata with Kale,	Cottage Cheese with Sliced	Strawberry and Chia

Day	Breakfast	Lunch	Dinner	Snack	Dessert
	Tomatoes and Basil		Potatoes, and Feta	Tomato and Cracked Pepper	Seed Pudding

Days 21 to 31

Day	Breakfast	Lunch	Dinner	Snack	Dessert
Day 21	Oatmeal with Sliced Pears and Almond Butter	Baked Trout with Walnut and Parsley Crust	Vegetarian Paella with Bell Peppers and Lima Beans	Greek Yogurt with Honey and Walnut	Coconut Rice Pudding
Day 22	Buckwheat Pancakes with Blueberry Compote	Spinach and Feta Stuffed Chicken Breast	Roasted Pork Tenderloin with Apples and Onions	Baked Kale Chips	Dark Chocolate and Avocado Mousse
Day 23	Scrambled Eggs with Spinach and Mushrooms	Pearl Barley Risotto with Asparagus and Lemon Zest	Wild Rice and Turkey Casserole	Almond and Date Energy Balls	Peach and Raspberry Crisp
Day 24	Quinoa Porridge with Apple and Cinnamon	Gazpacho with Fresh Cucumber and Bell Pepper	Grilled Turkey Burgers with Oatmeal and Herbs	Cottage Cheese with Sliced Tomato and Cracked Pepper	Lemon and Poppy Seed Loaf

Day	Breakfast	Lunch	Dinner	Snack	Dessert
Day 25	Smoothie Bowl with Banana, Kiwi, and Flaxseed	Lentil Soup with Carrots and Celery	Roasted Chicken with Root Vegetables	Apple Slices with Almond Butter	Grilled Pineapple with Honey and Mint
Day 26	Chia Pudding with Coconut Milk and Mango	Quinoa Tabbouleh with Cucumbers and Mint	Baked Haddock with a Crust of Herbs and Almonds	Spiced Roasted Chickpeas	Watermelon and Mint Sorbet
Day 27	Barley Breakfast Salad with Citrus and Walnuts	Grilled Chicken Salad with Mixed Greens and Avocado	Vegan Chili with Quinoa and Black Beans	Guacamole with Whole Grain Crackers	Baked Figs with Honey and Cream Cheese
Day 28	Whole Wheat Toast with Avocado and Poached Egg	Vegetable Stir-Fry with Tofu and Tamari Sauce	Zucchini Noodles with Tomato Sauce and Fresh Basil	Stuffed Cherry Tomatoes with Herbed Goat Cheese	Apricot and Pistachio Tart
Day 29	Baked Sweet Potato and Kale Hash	Stuffed Bell Peppers with Brown Rice and Herbs	Eggplant Parmesan Lightened Up	Banana and Oat Cookies	Chocolate Chip and Banana Muffins
Day 30	Millet Cereal with Raisins and Honey	Pan-Seared Cod with	Beef and Vegetable	Mixed Nuts and Dried	Vanilla Panna Cotta with

Day	Breakfast	Lunch	Dinner	Snack	Dessert
		Fennel and Orange Salad	Stew with Thyme	Fruit Trail Mix	Berry Compote
Day 31	Rice Cakes Topped with Ricotta and Fresh Berries	Butternut Squash Soup with a Hint of Ginger	Spinach and Mushroom Lasagna	Edamame with Sea Salt	Lemon and Poppy Seed Loaf

Stress Management Techniques for Seniors

Stress is a common factor that affects everyone, but it can be particularly challenging for seniors, especially those dealing with chronic conditions like diverticulitis. Managing stress is crucial because prolonged stress can exacerbate symptoms of many health issues, including digestive disorders. Fortunately, there are several effective strategies that seniors can adopt to reduce stress levels and improve their overall well-being.

One effective way to manage stress is through regular physical activity. Exercise not only keeps the body healthy but also releases endorphins, which are chemicals in the brain that act as natural painkillers and mood elevators. Seniors don't need to engage in intense workouts to get these benefits; even gentle activities like walking, tai chi, or yoga can significantly reduce stress levels. These activities are also great for maintaining flexibility, balance, and strength, which are essential for overall health in older age.

Another beneficial stress management technique is deep breathing exercises. These exercises are simple yet powerful tools that can help calm the mind and reduce tension in the body. By focusing on slow, deep breaths, seniors can trigger a relaxation response in the body, which helps lower heart rate and blood pressure, promoting a sense of calm. This practice can be done anywhere and anytime, making it an accessible option for stress relief.

Mindfulness and meditation are also excellent ways for seniors to manage stress. Mindfulness involves staying present and fully engaging with the here and now, which can help reduce anxiety caused by worrying about the future or dwelling on the past. Meditation, on the other hand, often involves sitting quietly and paying attention to thoughts, sounds, the sensations of breathing, or parts of the body. Both practices can help shift thoughts away from typical stressors, providing a break from the cycle of negative thoughts.

Social interaction is another critical aspect of stress management. Loneliness and isolation can lead to increased stress and depression, particularly among seniors. Engaging in social activities, whether it's joining a club, participating in group exercises, or simply spending time with family and friends, can provide significant emotional support and reduce stress. Laughter and companionship are known to increase serotonin levels, combatting feelings of depression and anxiety.

Gardening is a soothing activity that combines physical activity, mindfulness, and exposure to the outdoors and sunlight, which can help enhance mood and reduce feelings of stress. The act of caring for plants and watching them grow can provide a sense of purpose and accomplishment, which is particularly gratifying for seniors who may feel disconnected from their active roles in earlier life stages.

Music and art therapy can also be beautiful ways for seniors to express themselves and manage stress. Engaging in creative activities such as painting, drawing, playing music, or listening to favorite tunes can serve as a great distraction from stressors and help seniors explore new forms of expression and enjoyment.

Adequate sleep is essential for stress management. Poor sleep can exacerbate anxiety, irritability, and stress. Seniors should aim for 7-8 hours of quality sleep per night. Establishing a regular, calming bedtime routine can improve sleep quality significantly. This might include activities like reading, taking a warm bath, or listening to soft music.

Finally, seniors should consider talking to a counselor or therapist if they find it challenging to manage stress on their own. Professional help can provide tailored strategies to cope with stress based on individual needs. Therapists can also help address any underlying issues that might be contributing to increased stress levels, such as chronic health concerns, financial worries, or family dynamics.

By incorporating these strategies into their daily routines, seniors can significantly reduce their stress levels and improve their quality of life. Managing stress is not only about reducing the number of stressors in life but also about enhancing one's ability to handle the inevitable challenges that come with aging. With the right tools and support, seniors can protect their health and enjoy a more relaxed, joyful life.

Foods to Embrace and Avoid After 60

As individuals age, particularly after the age of 60, dietary needs change significantly, and this is even more pronounced for those managing conditions like diverticulitis. Digestive systems become more sensitive, requiring careful consideration of what to eat to maintain health and prevent discomfort. Understanding which foods to include and which to avoid is crucial for optimal digestive health and preventing flare-ups in seniors.

High-fiber foods are essential for seniors, especially those with diverticulitis because fiber helps to keep the digestive system flowing and prevents constipation, which can exacerbate diverticulitis symptoms. Whole grains such as oatmeal, whole wheat bread, brown rice, and barley provide the necessary fiber without being too harsh on the digestive system. Vegetables are excellent sources of vitamins, minerals, and fiber. Leafy greens like spinach, kale, and Swiss chard, along with cruciferous vegetables like broccoli and Brussels sprouts, should be cooked well to ease digestion. Fruits, particularly those with edible skins or seeds, offer significant fiber benefits. Apples, pears, and berries can be very beneficial and are best consumed cooked or as smoothies if digestion is a concern. Legumes, including beans, lentils, and chickpeas, offer both protein and fiber, making them excellent dietary staples. They should be well-cooked and blended into soups or purees for easier digestion.

Probiotic-rich foods support gut health by enhancing the beneficial bacteria in the digestive tract. These include yogurt and kefir with live active cultures and fermented vegetables like sauerkraut or kimchi, which should be consumed in moderation to avoid excess salt. Lean proteins are easier on the digestive system and reduce the workload on the gut. Good sources include poultry like chicken or turkey breasts without the skin, fish, particularly fatty types like salmon or mackerel that provide omega-3 fatty acids, which reduce inflammation, and eggs, which are generally easy to digest. Healthy fats are essential for overall health and help with the absorption of vitamins. Sources of healthy fats include avocados, nuts, and seeds, which should be chewed thoroughly or consumed as butter for easier digestion, and olive oil and other vegetable oils in moderation.

To prevent flare-ups and digestive discomfort, certain foods should be avoided, mainly if they have previously caused issues. High-fat and fried foods can increase the risk of constipation and exacerbate diverticulitis symptoms. This includes fried snacks, fast food, and anything cooked in excessive oil. Refined grains and sugar can disrupt the overall balance of the digestive system, leading to spikes in blood sugar and increased inflammation. These include white bread, pastries, and other products made from refined flour, sweets, and candies. Tough meats and processed meats can be difficult to digest and are often high in fats and preservatives.

Certain high-fiber foods can actually exacerbate problems if one has an active diverticulitis flare-up. These include raw vegetables with tough skins, corn, popcorn, and certain seeds and nuts. Lactose-containing foods can become problematic if seniors develop lactose intolerance, a common issue as lactase production decreases with age. This includes most dairy products, which need to be limited or avoided. Spicy foods and excess salt can irritate the digestive tract and should be consumed in moderation. Caffeine and alcohol can disrupt digestive functions and exacerbate symptoms of diverticulitis by stimulating the intestines and possibly leading to diarrhea or dehydration.

By tailoring their diet to include more beneficial foods and avoiding those that can cause harm, seniors can significantly improve their digestive health. This approach not only helps manage diverticulitis but also contributes to overall well-being and a better quality of life in later years. Regular consultations with healthcare providers and dietitians can further refine dietary choices to suit individual health needs and preferences.

Grocery Shopping Tips for Seniors

Navigating the grocery store and making healthful food choices can be a challenge, especially for seniors who must manage conditions like diverticulitis. As seniors aim to maintain a diet that supports their digestive health while minimizing flare-ups, it becomes imperative to shop smartly and efficiently. The following practical advice seeks to enhance the grocery shopping experience, ensuring seniors can choose the right foods and read labels effectively, making their trips to the store both more accessible and more effective.

Understanding the layout of the grocery store is the first step in effective shopping. Most stores are designed with fresh food sections along the perimeter; this includes produce, meats, and dairy items. Seniors should focus on these areas because fresh fruits, vegetables, and lean proteins are essential for a diverticulitis-friendly diet. Starting the shopping trip around the edge of the store ensures that the cart fills with nutrient-dense, fresh foods before reaching the inner aisles, where more processed foods are located.

When shopping for fruits and vegetables, it's beneficial to choose a variety of colors and types. Each color represents different nutrients and antioxidants that can help reduce inflammation and support overall health. For instance, leafy green vegetables like spinach and kale are high in fiber and vitamins, while berries are loaded with antioxidants that can help fight inflammation. Cooking these vegetables can make them easier to digest, which is particularly important for those managing diverticulitis.

For protein, lean meats such as chicken, turkey, and fish are excellent choices. These provide essential proteins without the extra fats that can exacerbate digestive issues. When selecting meat, it's crucial to look for labels that say "lean" or "extra lean" and to avoid processed meats like sausages or deli meats, which can contain additives and high levels of sodium. Fish, especially fatty types like salmon, are rich in omega-3 fatty acids, which are known for their anti-inflammatory properties.

Reading labels is a critical skill that every senior should develop. Nutritional labels provide essential information about the ingredients, nutritional content, and serving size of food items. Seniors should look for foods with high dietary fiber content while avoiding those high in fats and sugars. It's also important to watch for additives and preservatives that can irritate the digestive system. Ingredients are listed by quantity, from the highest to the lowest. This means that the first few ingredients make up the majority of what's in the product, so choosing products where sugars, fats, or artificial ingredients are not listed early can help maintain a healthier diet.

Another critical aspect of label reading is checking for sodium levels. A diet high in sodium can lead to water retention and high blood pressure, which is a concern for many seniors. Low-sodium products are preferable, especially for those with high blood pressure or kidney issues, which often accompany aging.

Seniors should also consider the practicality of food preparation. Opt for items that are easier to prepare and consume, especially for those with limited mobility or strength. For example, buying pre-cut fresh vegetables or fruits can save on prep time and make it easier to include these in meals. Similarly, choosing canned beans over dry ones can eliminate the need for prolonged soaking and cooking, which can be labor-intensive.

Organizational strategies can make grocery shopping more manageable. Creating a list before heading to the store helps seniors stay on track and avoid impulse buys that might not align with a diverticulitis-friendly diet. Organizing the list by store sections (produce, dairy, meats, and pantry items) can make the shopping trip quicker and more efficient. Some seniors might find it helpful to shop at quieter times to avoid the crowds and to take advantage of restocking days when fresh produce is most abundant.

Many grocery stores now offer services that can aid seniors in their shopping needs. Delivery services, curbside pickup, and senior discount days are options that can make shopping more accessible and more economical. For those who are tech-savvy, using online platforms to order groceries can be a convenient way to ensure they get the necessary items without the physical strain of a traditional shopping trip.

Incorporating these strategies into their shopping routine can help seniors manage their diverticulitis effectively while maintaining independence in their dietary choices. By focusing on nutrient-dense foods, learning to read and understand food labels, and utilizing available services, seniors can navigate the complexities of grocery shopping with confidence, ensuring they maintain a healthy, balanced diet that supports their digestive health and overall well-being.

CONCLUSION

Maintaining Your Dietary Gains

Maintaining a high-fiber diet and a healthy gut is crucial as you age, particularly for managing conditions like diverticulitis. A well-maintained diet not only supports digestive health but also enhances overall well-being, making it vital to sustain these dietary gains throughout the senior years. Implementing strategies that support consistent, healthful eating habits can help ensure that the benefits of a high-fiber diet are prolonged and that the digestive system remains robust.

First and foremost, establishing a routine is beneficial. Consistency in eating times and the types of food consumed can help regulate digestive processes and reinforce healthy gut flora. As seniors, sticking to a regular eating schedule helps the body to process and absorb nutrients efficiently and can reduce the likelihood of digestive discomfort. It's also helpful to plan meals ahead of time. Weekly meal planning can ensure that the diet remains rich in fiber and low in processed foods, which often lack nutritional value and can aggravate digestive issues.

Incorporating a variety of fiber-rich foods into the diet is vital to sustaining dietary gains. This variety ensures that all types of necessary fibers are consumed. Soluble fiber, found in oats, apples, and beans, helps to soften stool, which can prevent the straining that exacerbates diverticulitis. Insoluble fiber, found in whole grains and vegetables, adds bulk to stool and helps food pass more quickly through the stomach and intestines. Eating a diverse range of fruits, vegetables, and whole grains also provides a broad spectrum of nutrients and antioxidants, supporting overall health beyond just the digestive system.

Hydration plays a critical role in maintaining digestive health, especially when consuming a high-fiber diet. Fiber works best when it absorbs water, which bulks up the stool and allows for smoother passage through the intestines.

Seniors should drink adequate fluids throughout the day. Water is the best choice; however, other fluids like herbal teas can contribute to daily hydration needs without adding excessive calories or sugars.

Regular physical activity is another crucial component of sustaining a healthy gut. Exercise helps accelerate the transit time of food through the colon and reduces the time the body is exposed to potential toxins in the stool. Gentle activities, such as walking or yoga, can be particularly beneficial for seniors, helping to maintain mobility and reduce stress, which can also impact digestive health.

Continued education about nutrition can empower seniors to make informed choices about their diet. Understanding which foods enhance gut health and which might lead to flare-ups can help in making better dietary decisions. This knowledge can also evolve as nutritional science advances, so staying informed about the latest research can be incredibly beneficial.

For seniors managing diverticulitis, it's also essential to monitor the diet closely and adjust it based on the body's reactions. Keeping a food diary can be an effective way to track which foods contribute to symptoms and which foods seem to support well-being. This diary can be a valuable resource for discussions with healthcare providers about how to continue best-managing diverticulitis through diet.

Engaging with healthcare providers for regular check-ups can help seniors adjust their diets according to their changing health needs. As the body ages, its ability to digest certain foods can change, and diet adjustments may be necessary to accommodate decreased stomach acid levels or altered gut motility.

Finally, building a support network can also aid in maintaining these dietary gains. Sharing meals with friends or family, joining groups with similar health interests, or participating in cooking classes can reinforce positive nutritional habits. Social interactions can also provide emotional support, which is crucial for overall health and can influence eating habits and digestive health.

By integrating these strategies into everyday life, seniors can sustain their dietary gains, maintaining a high-fiber diet that supports a healthy gut and overall well-being as they age. These habits not only help manage conditions like diverticulitis but also contribute to a more vibrant, active, and healthy lifestyle in the golden years.

Thank you for completing "Diverticulitis Diet After 60." We hope that you have found the strategies and recipes beneficial for managing your health. Sharing your overall experience and the impact this book has had on your dietary habits would greatly help us and inspire others.

How You Can Share Your Review:

Through Amazon.com:

- Go to the Amazon page where you found my book.

- Navigate to the 'Customer Reviews' section.

- Click on 'Write a customer review' to share your valuable insights.

Instant QR Code Access: Simply scan the QR code below with your smartphone to be directed to the Amazon review section.